Other titles in this series:

THE BEST IN TENT CAMPING

A GUIDE FOR CAR CAMPERS WHO HATE RVs,
CONCRETE SLABS, AND LOUD PORTABLE STEREOS

NORTHERN CALIFORNIA

FOURTH EDITION

BILL MAI
Revised by Cindy Coloma

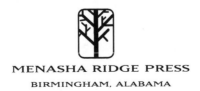

MENASHA RIDGE PRESS
BIRMINGHAM, ALABAMA

*To Mom and Dad, who gave me a love of mountain air
and an appreciation of dusty roads.
And to my son, Cody Martinusen—outdoorsman extraordinaire.*
—Cindy Coloma

Copyright © 2008 by Cindy Coloma and Bill Mai
All rights reserved
Printed in the United States of America
Published by Menasha Ridge Press
Distributed by Publishers Group West
Fourth edition, second printing 2010

Library of Congress Cataloging-in-Publication Data

Coloma, Cindy.
 The best in tent, camping northern California: a guide for car campers who hate RVs, concrete
slabs, and loud portable stereos/Cindy Coloma with Bill Mai. —4th ed.
     p. cm.
 Rev. ed. of: The best in tent camping, northern California/Hans Huber. 3rd. ed. c2004.
 Includes index.
 ISBN-13: 978-0-89732-674-2
 ISBN-10: 0-89732-674-1
 1. Campsites, facilities, etc.—California, Northern—Guidebooks. 2. Camping—California, Northern—
Guidebooks. 3. California, Northern—Guidebooks. I. Huber, Hans, 1964— Best in tent camping,
northern California. II. Title.
 GV191.42.C2C67 2008
 917.9404'54—dc22

                    2008037018

Cover and text design by Ian Szymkowiak, Palace Press International, Inc.
Cover photo by Jordan Summers
Cartography by Steve Jones
Indexing by Cynthia J. Coan

Menasha Ridge Press
P.O. Box 43673
Birmingham, Alabama 35243
www.menasharidge.com

TABLE OF CONTENTS

THE SIERRA NEVADA 103

YOSEMITE   153

SHASTA-TRINITY   173

PREFACE

WHY DO WE LOVE CAMPING? Some people don't understand it. And how can we explain why civilized people find it thrilling to pack up their cars with what's already in their houses—beds, shelter, food, water, games—to venture into nature to cook, clean, eat, sleep, play, and explore?

Perhaps it's some ancestral instinct or primal call that draws us to live and play within the wilds, if only for a time. Or maybe it's because nothing tastes better than pancakes on a paper plate with a cup of piping coffee on a chilly mountain morn, or a half-charred hot dog or marshmallow cooked over a smoky campfire.

Every July, one of my closest of friends, Michelle (LaCom) Ower, travels with her husband and kids to congregate with extended family at a primitive Trinity Forest campground for two or three weeks. They've been doing it every single year, in the same place, since the 1960s. Sometimes my family and I join them, and I'm ever amazed at their three generations of people, camping gear, and stories—or at the neighboring campers who have become lifelong friends and also annually camp beside the LaCom/Owers. It's tradition, it's often where the strongest memories are made, it's a home beneath the pines that's every bit a part of them as their houses in Tennessee, the Bay Area, and northern Oregon. Whatever the reasons, we, young and old, love to camp. It can't be explained and we need not try—those who love it, simply do.

And so, this book is here to help answer that call and to provide a complete guide to make the plan become reality. The 55 campgrounds in five regions of Northern California offer a great diversity in elevation, geography, size, and amenities. Each campground is rated in categories of beauty, site privacy, spaciousness, quiet, security, and cleanliness.

I've lived in Northern California since I was 7 years old, and as a child, my parents took me camping and backpacking all over the region from the coast to the many mountain ranges and wilderness areas. The camping bug stuck, and now my children are reaching toward adulthood with their own great love of the outdoors. And though I have traveled all over the world and the United States, I'm still continually surprised and awed by what I discover or find anew right here in my own backyard—because Northern California offers an unending display of rugged mountains, savage coastlines, and the captivating beauty of lakes, rivers, valleys, and gentle coves.

So where do you want to go? What kind of activities do you prefer? Are you seeking high mountains with hot showers or a lake view *au naturel?* There's a campground and region to fit every interest and to satisfy every outdoor dream. You can fill your trip with activities or keep it relaxing and low key.

And yet, even with this guide, you can never guess what you'll discover until you venture out. Maybe you'll meet the LaCom/Owers on their annual trip, or see wildlife you've only encountered on the television screen, or you'll grow closer to your children and grandchildren simply by making s'mores and telling stories beside a campfire. Or you may discover a vastness of eternity and an unparalleled wonder beneath the brightest stars you've ever seen.

We don't know what we'll find, or what will find us, but it's sure to be. Then we'll take the experiences back to our cities and towns and civilized lives. And we'll plan for the next trip. Because this is why we love camping.

—Cindy Coloma

THE BEST
IN TENT
CAMPING

A GUIDE FOR CAR CAMPERS WHO HATE RVs, CONCRETE SLABS, AND LOUD PORTABLE STEREOS

NORTHERN CALIFORNIA

FOURTH EDITION

INTRODUCTION

CAMP **N**ORTHERN **C**ALIFORNIA. Drive up Interstate 5 and feel the big granite block of the Sierra Nevada looming to the east, 400 miles long. Ahead, in the Shasta-Trinities, is Mount Shasta, 14,161 feet high and topped with snow. To the west is the Coast Range, an ocean of sharp mountains and redwoods dipping down into the Pacific, where the white-blue waves break on rocky shores. From Lassen Volcanic National Park north, the Cascade Range is all volcanic, up past Alturas to Lava Beds National Monument. The weather is as wild as the land. Nowhere else can you feel so remote, camp on such wild, beautiful land, and fish untamed rivers running to the sea.

GEOGRAPHY

For the purposes of this book, Northern California is everything above a line drawn from Santa Cruz across to Yosemite National Park and the Nevada border and north to the Oregon border. This area is divided into the Coast Range, the Cascade Range, the Sierra Nevada, Yosemite, and Shasta-Trinity.

The Coast Range includes the hundreds of miles of rock cliffs, sandy coves, and beaches between Santa Cruz and Oregon, as well as the mountains running down to the sea. The Shasta-Trinity region of California extends from the top of the Sacramento Valley north to Oregon until it reaches a handshake toward the coastal ranges. East of I-5 is the Cascade Range in the north, the Modoc plateau, and Lassen Volcanic National Park, where the Cascade Range runs south and merges with the Sierra Nevada and then south into the wonderland that is Yosemite.

WHERE TO GO AND WHEN

Depending upon elevation and location, great camping in Northern California can be found from May to October, and even year-round. Camping in the mountains is mostly for late spring, summer, and early fall. The Sierra Nevada, Cascade, Yosemite, and Shasta-Trinity climate is fairly reliable as soon as the winter snow pack melts. But until summer fully arrives, watch the weather. It can get bone cold in the higher regions even in the summer.

Summer heat (June to mid-September) can be sweltering at lower elevations, especially in the Cascades and Shasta-Trinity. This is the perfect time to spend the afternoons on the lake after a morning exploring waterfalls and caves. Or pack your gear and escape the heat at those high mountain campgrounds that can be enjoyed only a few months out of the year.

The Coast can be explored anytime, but it's especially pleasant from September to November for less fog and more sunshine. The coastal climate is an inconsistent tyrant

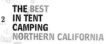

the rest of the year, but those sunshiny days quickly dry the memories of those filled with rain and fog. Enjoy the sun, it may be gone within hours or hang around for days—neither you nor the weatherman can guess which.

Some mountain campgrounds in Northern California are open even in the winter for the hardy breed who want to snow-camp. Watch the weather, come prepared, and let a few people know you're there—including a local ranger station.

THE RATING SYSTEM

The 55 best campgrounds are rated in various categories—five stars is best, and one star is acceptable. Use the rating system to select the wonderful campground that combines the elements that best suit you.

BEAUTY

Although all 55 campgrounds in this book are beautiful, some are absolutely sensational, and these rate five stars. Mountains, streams, waterfalls, and sunsets all conspire for a drop-dead campground personality. One- to four-star campgrounds are no dogs, either, but possess a less-spectacular beauty that will grow on you.

PRIVACY

Some campgrounds are beautifully built. The sites are arranged to take maximum advantage of the contour of the land, and the vegetation gives each one the most privacy possible. Good architecture cuts down on the cringe factor when other campers pull in next door. A bit of privacy makes you feel at home from the moment you step out of your car. What a difference!

SPACIOUSNESS

I want flat land to pitch a tent on. And I want the flat area far enough from the picnic table so my camping mate can make coffee without waking me, and far enough from the fire pit that the embers don't burn little holes in the tent. And I want a view. A view from each campsite is part of the spacious feeling that qualifies a campground for five stars in this category.

QUIET

Quiet is part of beautiful. There's nothing like the sound of a generator or a boom box to ruin a beautiful campsite. I consider white noise such as the roar of a river to raise the quiet rating, since it is a natural noise and drowns out the sounds of other campers.

SECURITY

Most of the campsites in the top 55 have campground hosts that keep a good eye on the property, which makes the campground safer than a good neighborhood. The farther the campground is from an urban center, the more secure it is. Often, you can leave your valuables with the hosts if you're going to be gone for a day or so, but don't leave little things lying around. A blue jay will take off with a pair of sunglasses, and you never can tell what a visiting bear will decide has food value.

CLEANLINESS

Most campgrounds in the top 55 are well tended. Sometimes, on big weekends, places can get a little rank—not unlike one's kitchen after a big party. I appreciate the little things, like the campground host who came around with a rake after each site was vacated to police the place. That particular campground received five stars in the cleanliness department.

GOOD PLANNING

A little planning makes a good camping trip great. First, decide where and when you want to go. Then, phone that district's Ranger Headquarters to make sure the campground is open and has water. See if the ranger recommends other campgrounds. See if it's going to be busy. If it is, reserve ahead if possible. All national-forest campgrounds must be reserved at least ten days in advance. Remember, if you arrive and don't like the reserved site, the campground host will move you if another site is available.

Next, get your equipment together. Everybody knows what basics to bring tent camping. A tent (of course), the sleeping bags, a cooler, a stove, pots, utensils, a water jug, matches, a can opener, and so forth. But it's those little things that you suddenly wish you had that make for a really happy camper. The number one objective is a good night's sleep.

Bring earplugs. You need earplugs to get a good snooze. The first night or two out camping, the unfamiliar flap of the tent drives you crazy if you don't have earplugs. Also, a snoring mate sleeping a foot away from you is nighttime hell on earth without earplugs. In addition, earplugs block out all that night nature stuff that interferes with a righteous camper's Z's.

Don't forget to pack your own pillow. A good pillow gets your shoulders off the deck and lets your hips and behind take the weight. Use your clothes bag as an additional pillow (consider inflatable pillows sold at camping stores). Bring a thin foam mattress or buy those self-inflating pads. Buy a Spidermat—a device that keeps your pad from slipping on the tent floor and keeps your sleeping bag on top of it. Air mattresses are okay but susceptible to puncture. Never buy a double air mattress—every time your mate moves you'll get tossed around. Get a sleeping bag that is good and warm. Nothing is worse than being cold at night, and no sleeping bag is too warm. Just bring a sheet so you can sleep under it at first, then crawl into the bag when it gets nippy. Check the weather. If it's going to be cold, remember to bring socks and sweatpants to sleep in. A sweatshirt with a hood is invaluable, since you lose a lot of heat through your head.

Bring a water bottle from which to drink at night. Consequently, a pee jar (a pee pot for ladies) just outside the tent is a great idea. You can stumble outside, use it, and empty it in the toilet in the morning.

Nothing disturbs your Z's like grit inside the tent, so bring something to put outside the tent to clean your feet on. In the woods, a square of AstroTurf works fine. At the seashore or in the desert, a tray full of water in which to dip your feet works best. Bring a small brush for sweeping up whatever grit leaks in.

Remember flashlights. The mini-MagLites work okay, and if you take off the lens, you can hang them from a tent loop and actually read. Be careful since the little bulb can get damn hot and will burn fabric or fingers. What works even better is a head lamp. You can buy them at any outdoor store. Just strap the lamp around your head with an adjustable elastic band. Everywhere you look, there's light. They're great for finding stuff, cleaning up in the dark after dinner, and reading. And remember duct tape. "If you can't fix it, duct-tape it" is a camping maxim.

Bring a sponge to clean off the picnic table. A plastic tablecloth is nice, too (bring little pushpins to secure it so it won't blow away). A plastic bowl or a blow-up sink from Basic Designs (around $9 at Sportmart) is invaluable for washing dishes. Picnic table benches get mighty hard, so bring a cushion. Buy a cheap lawn chair, and get the inexpensive umbrella that attaches to the back of the chair, so you can sit around the camp out of the sun. While sitting around, you'll want a fly swatter to wreak revenge on a lazy droning fly or two, and mosquito repellent for that irksome gnat in your ear. Bring a little leaf rake to police your camp area. Remember binoculars, a bird book, and a wildflower book, so you can put a name to what you see.

Good water jugs are those two-and-a-half-gallon plastic jobs sold in supermarkets. On most of them, you can twist off the top and refill them. They travel best with their valves up to avoid any leakage. Take a hot shower. Basic Designs (and other outfits) sells a solar shower bag that really works. After a day in the sun sitting on a hot rock, the water will be deliciously hot! Or bring along nonscented diaper wipes for a quick sponge bath. They work.

Don't be afraid to ask fellow campers for help or for stuff you might have forgotten. All campers know what it's like to forget basic stuff and love to help fellow campers. There's always a mechanic on vacation camping at the next site over when your car won't start, or somebody with extra white gas for your stove. Think heartily about your fellow campers. Wave and say "Hi." And be sure to return the favor if your fellow camper has forgotten something.

The campfire is an important camp event. Stores around the campground sell bundles of wood, and often the campground host sells wood. Also, there may be windfalls around the campground from which you can take wood (ask the campground host). You need a good camp saw for that. An absolute essential is a can of charcoal starter fluid. This guarantees a fire even in a driving rain. Naturally, don't forget chocolate, graham crackers, and marshmallows for roasting.

Fix up your car before you go. Nothing can be a bigger bummer than a mechanical breakdown on your way out. Have a mechanic check your water hoses and the air pressure in your tires before you load up. Remember, your car will be loaded down with stuff, and this will put a strain on your tires and cooling system. Bring an extra fan belt. Nothing can shut down the car like a snapped fan belt that you have to special-order from Japan. Even if you don't know a fan belt from third base, bring one. Somebody will come along who knows how to install it. Make sure your spare tire is correctly inflated. Mishap #999 is when you put on your spare, let the car down, and find out the spare is flat.

If you fish, be sure to get a license and display it. Fishing without a license is a misdemeanor, punishable by a maximum fine of $1,000 and/or six months in jail. On your way into the campground, stop at a local store and find out what the folks are using for bait. Buy it. This will save you a lot of experimentation and probably provide you with a good meal.

Remember the bears. Never leave your cooler out. Put it in the trunk or disguise it with a blanket if you have a hatchback or a van. Don't eat in your tent. Take all cosmetics, soap, and other scented products and put them in the car; disguise them too. A bear will rip off a car door to get to a tube of lip balm. Bring a small bottle of bleach to wipe down the picnic table at night. Bears don't like bleach (but don't put too much faith in this!). If a bear raids your camp looking for food, beat on pots and pans and shoo it away like you would a naughty dog. So don't worry—even the boldest of bears won't dream of going into a tent unless it smells food inside.

Don't forget about mosquitoes. Where you have rain, trees, and rivers, there are mosquitoes—and they're hungry. Bring a couple of different kinds of repellent since there are 3,000 kinds of mosquitoes. Repellent some mosquitoes detest others find very attractive. I like 3M's Ultrathon repellent—this is serious stuff. And, sometimes, Avon's Skin-So-Soft works wonders. Other times, it draws mosquitoes from miles away. A great idea if you are going to camp for a couple days is a screen house. You can set it up over the picnic table or in a sunny spot and lounge in there while less-prepared neighbors are under siege. Coleman sells a lighter-duty one for just over $100—Eureka sells a sturdier, larger one for, of course, many more bucks.

Think about swimming. Bring old tennis shoes or buy water booties for wading in streams and in lakes. Goggles are cool to check out what the trout are doing. Bring any rubber flotation device you can afford and carry in your auto that will get your highly vulnerable body on the gorgeous blue mountain lakes but definitely out of the frigid water. Think air mattress with an air pump driven off the cigarette lighter of the car. They are lightweight and fun. Be careful not to set your device down on sharp shale or pine needles—and come prepared with a repair kit.

Think about dispersed camping. With a fire permit, a shovel, and a bucket of water, you can camp just about anywhere in the national forests (consult the Ranger District Headquarters). The fire permit costs nothing, and there are miles and miles of fire roads and lumber roads you can explore to find the dispersed campground of your dreams.

SETTLING IN

When you come into a campground, be aware of a certain psychological barrier. This is a new place. Suddenly, you've driven all this way, and the campground doesn't look that hot. You feel disappointed. You feel like the new kid at school. The other campers look up from their game of gin rummy and hope you won't camp next to them as you drive around the campground loops and look helplessly at the open sites. Nothing looks good enough.

Park your car. Pull into the first available site that could possibly do. Then walk around the campground. You have half an hour to decide before you pick your site and pay. Once you get out and walk, you'll break through that "new kid at school" dilemma and soon feel like you're a part of the place. It's odd. Suddenly, you don't mind camping next to the gin rummy players. You realize that this is your campground as well as theirs. By the next morning, the whole place will feel like home, and the gin rummy players will seem like the best of neighbors. You won't understand why you didn't immediately recognize this campground as the best of all campgrounds.

When you plan a camping trip, try to stay in one campground for at least three days. Stay one day, and you end up spending most of your time packing and unpacking and getting familiar with the campground. Stay three days, and you'll relax and have fun.

Go tent camping. Live in paradise for a few days. Camping makes you want to sin like the damned, sleep like the righteous, and hike like the last of the great American walkers. It's a balm for the weary soul!

ANIMAL AND PLANT HAZARDS

SNAKES   Northern California has a variety of snakes—including gopher snakes, king snakes, and racers—most of which are benign. Rattlesnakes are the exception, and they dwell in every area of the state: mountains, foothills, valleys, and deserts. The most common species found in the north of the state are the Northern Pacific rattlesnake and the Western diamondback. The whole of California has the sidewinder, the speckled rattlesnake, the red diamond rattlesnake, the Southern Pacific rattlesnake, the Great Basin rattlesnake, and the Mojave rattlesnake, according to the California Department of Fish and Game.

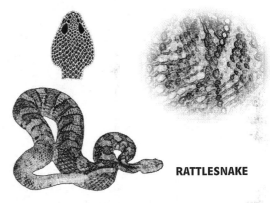

RATTLESNAKE

When hiking, stick to well-used trails, and wear over-the-ankle boots and loose-fitting long pants. Rattlesnakes like to bask in the sun when it's cooler and rest in the shade when it's hot (including rocks, near water, beneath picnic tables). They won't bite unless surprised or threatened. Do not step or put your hands where you cannot see, and avoid wandering around in the dark. Step on logs and rocks, never over them, and be especially careful when climbing rocks or gathering firewood. Always avoid walking through dense brush or willow thickets. Hibernation season is November through February.

TICKS   Ticks are often found on brush and tall grass waiting to hitch a ride on a warm-blooded passerby. They are most active between April and October. Among the local varieties of ticks, the Western black-legged tick is the primary carrier of Lyme disease. To reduce your chances of ticks getting under your skin, wear light-colored clothing so ticks can be spotted before they make it to the skin. Most important, be sure to visually check your hair, back of neck, armpits, and socks at the end of the hike. During your posthike shower, take a moment to do a more complete body check. For ticks that are already embedded, removal with tweezers is best. Use disinfectant solution on the wound.

POISON OAK   Poison oak is rampant in the shady canyons and riparian woodlands of Northern California. It grows in moist areas, favoring shade trees and water sources.

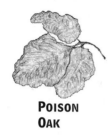

POISON OAK

Avoiding contact is the most effective way to prevent the painful, itchy rashes associated with these plants. Identify the plant by its three-leaf structure, with two leaves on opposite sides of the stem and one extending from the center. Refrain from scratching because bacteria under fingernails can cause infection. Wash and dry the rash thoroughly, applying calamine lotion to help dry out the rash. If you do come in contact with one of these plants, remember that oil-contaminated clothes, pets, or hiking gear can easily cause an irritating rash on you or someone else, so wash not only any exposed parts of your body but also clothes, gear, and pets if applicable.

GPS CAMPGROUND-ENTRANCE COORDINATES

Readers can easily access all campgrounds in this book by using the directions given, the overview map, and the trail maps, which show at least one major road leading into the area. But for those who enjoy using the latest GPS technology to navigate, the necessary data has been provided. For readers who own a GPS unit, the UTM coordinates provided with the campground profile may be entered into the GPS unit. Just make sure your GPS unit is set to navigate using the UTM system in conjunction with WGS84 datum.

UTM COORDINATES

The GPS data for each hike includes zone, easting, and northing numbers, in addition to latitude and longitude. Here's an example from Butano State Park Campground (page 21):

UTM Zone (WGS84) 10S
Easting 0557474
Northing 4119249

The zone number (10S) refers to one of the 60 longitudinal (vertical) zones of a map using the Universal Transverse Mercator (UTM) projection. Each zone is 6 degrees wide. The zone letter (S) refers to one of the 20 latitudinal (horizontal) zones that span from 80° south to 84° north. The easting number (0557474) references in meters how far east the point is from the zero value for eastings, which runs north–south through Greenwich, England. Increasing easting coordinates on a topo map or on your GPS screen indicate that you are moving east; decreasing easting coordinates indicate that you are moving west.

In the northern hemisphere, the northing number (4119249) references in meters how far you are from the equator. Above the equator, northing coordinates increase by 1,000 meters between each parallel line of latitude (east–west lines). On a topo map or GPS receiver, increasing northing numbers indicate that you are traveling north; decreasing northing coordinates indicate that you are traveling south.

BILL MAI

Bill's mother was an avid camper, and she developed in her son a love for the outdoors. Inspired by the Native American "digs" that his mother worked on in the Denver Museum of Natural History and their many camping jaunts to Maine, the Adirondacks, and numerous locations in the West, Bill continued to foster his enthusiasm for camping.

Driven by his sense of adventure, Bill did a stint in Pernambuco, Brazil, after college, working for the Peace Corps on a small rancher's cooperative. Reminiscent of 1830s New Mexico, there were no cars and no electricity but an abundance of cattle drives and gunfights in the streets.

After shaking off the chaps and spurs, Bill donned the vestments of academia to teach at several colleges around London. In the interim, he composed several short stories and a novel. Unwilling to give up his roots, he continued to camp in England, biking down old county lanes and camping in farming fields.

Now Bill continues to write screenplays and wonderful books about his love of camping, including *The Best in Tent Camping: Southern California,* the series counterpart to this book. And, of course, he continues to travel extensively on camping and fishing expeditions around Baja California and California proper.

CINDY COLOMA

While Cindy was growing up, her parents often took her and her sister exploring the mountains of the western states and driving dirt roads to "see where they went." She's camped in old campers, truck beds, tents, primitive cabins, the backseat of a Volkswagen bug, and sleeping bags beneath the stars.

She has passed her love of the outdoors down to her children, especially her oldest son, who wanted to try surviving in the Yolla-Bolly Wilderness (his favorite area) for his high-school senior project. Early snows dampened the idea, however, and Cindy was relieved though she was proud of his adventurous spirit.

Cindy is the author of several novels (written under the name Cindy Martinusen) set in Northern California, Europe, and Southeast Asia. She enjoys exploring the regions of her research firsthand, taking in the cultures and landscapes. But home is most sweet, and since she was 7 years old Cindy has lived in the Redding area. She continues to live there with her husband, Nieldon, and their three children.

Cindy continues to write both fiction and nonfiction while also working with published and aspiring writers on their projects. She and her family regularly enjoy the many outdoor wonders and activities found in Northern California. For more information about Cindy, visit her Web site, **www.cindycoloma.com.**

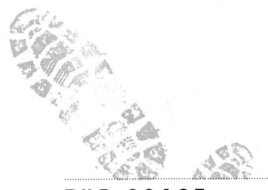

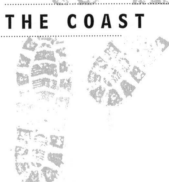

THE COAST

01
ALBEE CREEK CAMPGROUND

DRIVE 5 MILES OFF US 101 on Mattole Road through incredible stands of redwoods (use daytime headlights) and come to Albee Creek Campground 0.3 miles up an access road on the right. This beautiful campground is framed by Albee Creek on the east and Bull Creek to the south—most of the campsites nestle at the base of a forested hillside to the north. This is nice open camping for folks who don't want the "darkness at noon" aspect of the redwood forest. Down below on the little prairie is an old fruit orchard planted by John Albee, who carried mail into Bull Valley in the old days before the forest became Humboldt Redwoods State Park.

From Albee Campground, catch the Big Trees–Albee Creek Loop Trail. This is a 2.5-mile round-trip hike that follows Albee Creek east as it meanders just south of Mattole Road through the Rockefeller Forest, the world's largest grove of old-growth redwood. The average age of these trees falls between 500 and 1,200 years, with the oldest-known tree at 2,200 years old. Many measure more than 300 feet high, with some topping 360 feet. Hike under these trees among the calypso orchids, fetid adder's tongues, and redwood sorrel, and think about what the trees meant to the Native Americans in this region. They used them to make dugout canoes, plank and bark houses, and furniture. The shredded inner bark was made into women's skirts.

The first strangers to see the redwoods were the Chinese more than 2,000 years ago. Accounts tell of a junk captain, Hee-li, who followed his compass in the direction he thought was east (what did he think when he saw the sun setting in the east instead of the west?). Four months later he landed in a place with wonderful weather and gigantic trees with thick, reddish bark. Hee-li checked out his compass and found a small

> *Come out of the Big Trees into the sunshine at this pretty little spot.*

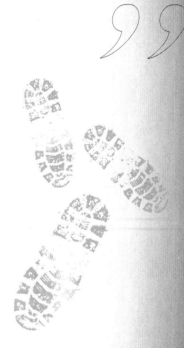

RATINGS

Beauty: ✪ ✪ ✪ ✪ ✪
Privacy: ✪ ✪ ✪
Spaciousness: ✪ ✪ ✪ ✪
Quiet: ✪ ✪ ✪
Security: ✪ ✪ ✪ ✪ ✪
Cleanliness: ✪ ✪ ✪ ✪

KEY INFORMATION

ADDRESS: Albee Creek Campground Humboldt Redwoods State Park P.O. Box 100 Weott, CA 95571

OPERATED BY: California State Parks

INFORMATION: (707) 946-2409; www.parks.ca.gov or www.humboldt redwoods.org

OPEN: May–mid-October

SITES: 22 sites for tents, 18 for tents or RVs

EACH SITE HAS: Picnic table, fireplace, food locker

ASSIGNMENT: Reservations online or by phone, assigned by ranger

REGISTRATION: At entrance; reserve by phone, (800) 444-7275, or online, www.reserve america.com

FACILITIES: Water, flush toilets, coin-operated showers, wood for sale, wheelchair-accessible sites

PARKING: At individual site

FEE: $20; $7.50 nonrefundable reservation fee

ELEVATION: 320 feet

RESTRICTIONS: *Pets:* Dogs on leash only, in campground
Fires: In fireplace
Alcohol: No restrictions
Vehicles: RVs up to 33 feet
Other: 14-day stay limit (7 in summer); reservations recommended on holidays and summer weekends, otherwise first come, first served

cockroach wedged under the needle. Upon removal of the cockroach, the needle swung around, and Hee-li sailed back home to China.

Next came the Spanish missionaries, who saw the redwoods near Monterey and cut them for roof beams in the missions. They soon realized that *Palo colorado* had wonderful properties. Father Junipero Serra had his coffin made of redwood. A century later his exhumed coffin was in perfect condition.

Then Dr. Josiah Gregg and a group of forty-niners came through these parts and discovered Humboldt Bay (which he named after his hero, Alexander von Humboldt, the 19th-century German scientist, naturalist, and geographer). Gold was discovered on the Trinity and the Klamath rivers. Forty-niners flooded north in 1850, and Humboldt County, with its wonderful bay and bountiful redwoods, was on its way to being the most populated region on the northern coast.

A big draw in the park is the Eel River, with springtime canoeing and the wildflower bloom. Hike down along the Eel. Pick up the River Trail where the Big Trees–Albee Creek Trail loops back around near the Rockefeller Loop. From here, the River Trail heads down the west side of the Eel to the Children's Forest, where a stone marker records the names of local children who died in the early 1900s. The fire-hollowed trees here once were goose pens. The round-trip just tops 5 miles.

As tame as Albee Creek, Bull Creek, and the Eel River look in the summer and fall, think twice. In 1955 and 1964 there were monster floods here. On the way from Garberville on US 101, look for the markers far above the highway that record the level of the raging water at the height of the flood. In 1955, near Albee Campground, Bull Creek raged through the town of Bull Creek, taking out 35 houses and the cemetery. Later, coffins were found in the branches of redwoods in the Rockefeller Forest.

Drive west on Mattole Road to Panther Gap (elevation 2,477 feet) and look over the watershed that these creeks and river service. When excessive logging cleared away the trees, there was nothing to stop the rain running off the slopes. The locals are thus caught

MAP

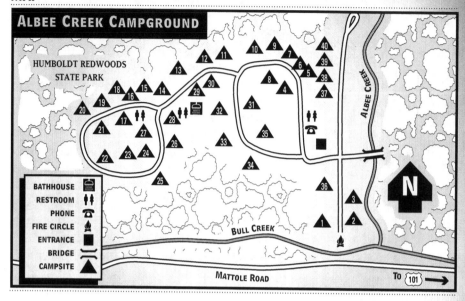

ALBEE CREEK CAMPGROUND

HUMBOLDT REDWOODS
STATE PARK

BATHHOUSE
RESTROOM
PHONE
FIRE CIRCLE
ENTRANCE
BRIDGE
CAMPSITE

ALBEE CREEK

BULL CREEK

MATTOLE ROAD

To 101

N

on the horns of a dilemma: many work for the lumber companies, but none of them want to see their houses swept away when the floods come.

Continue over Panther Gap down to the picturesque little hamlet of Honeydew (named for the sweet-tasting aphid dew beneath cottonwoods down by the river). There's good fishing on the Mattole River between Honeydew and Petrolia, home of the Hideaway Bar and Grill near the Lindley Bridge. They have delicious cinnamon rolls and hamburgers.

Humboldt Redwoods State Park has huge trees and huge mosquitoes in the late spring and summer—prepare!

GETTING THERE

From Weott north of Garberville, drive 2 miles north to Mattole Road, then drive west 5 miles to the Albee Creek Campground entrance on the right. Go 0.3 miles up the access road to the campground.

GPS COORDINATES

UTM Zone (WGS84) 10T

Easting 0414282

Northing 4467410

Latitude N 40° 21' 10.2530"

Longtitude W 124° 0' 33.8542"

02

BIG BASIN REDWOODS STATE PARK CAMPGROUNDS

> *Good tent camping, tent cabins, great hiking, marbled murrelets, and it's near Santa Cruz.*

THIS PARK IS THE GRANDDADDY of all the incredible California state parks. Big Basin has wonderful camping, as well as tent cabins with interior wood stoves. Lovely Wastahi Campground is all walk-in tent campsites, with the farthest campsite 200 feet from the parking areas. Huckleberry is all walk-in as well, with the farthest site 50 feet from the parking. With Blooms Campground and Sempervirens Campground, Big Basin has another 102 developed campsites for RVs, but the park doesn't feel at all crowded. The huge redwoods give Big Basin a certain eerie calm.

On May 15, 1900, Andrew P. Hill camped at the base of Slippery Rock with 50 other conservationists. Together they formed the Sempervirens Club. Named for the *Sequoia sempervirens,* or redwood, the club was able to fend off the lumbermen and promote the creation of California's first state park from a deed of 3,800 acres of primeval forest. Now Big Basin has 16,000 ocean-facing acres of Santa Cruz Mountain full of redwoods, Douglas fir, knob-cone pine, oak, marsh, and chaparral, thanks to the Save the Redwoods League and the Sempervirens Fund.

To get to know Big Basin, you have to hike or mountain bike. Driving an automobile in these mountain areas is chiefly a white-knuckle blur of naked fear, brake lights, and squealing tires. Pull over, park the car, and put on your hiking boots.

First, take the little Redwood Nature Trail loop to pay respects to an ancient redwood grove on the flat above Opal Creek. Look for azaleas blooming in early summer and pick huckleberries in August. You'll see Big Basin's tallest tree, the 329-foot Mother of the Forest, the big-girthed Father of the Forest, and the Chimney Tree. Mother's roots pull 500 gallons of water up from the ground, which she releases as moisture into the air—no wonder the forest is dank and lush.

RATINGS

Beauty: ☆ ☆ ☆ ☆ ☆
Privacy: ☆ ☆ ☆ ☆
Spaciousness: ☆ ☆ ☆ ☆
Quiet: ☆ ☆ ☆
Security: ☆ ☆ ☆ ☆ ☆
Cleanliness: ☆ ☆ ☆ ☆

Another quick hike is up the Sequoia Trail to Sempervirens Falls. The trailhead is right by Park Headquarters, and the trail is signed for Sempervirens Falls on the way up and Park Headquarters on the way back. The forest floor is bedded with ferns, and in the spring you'll see trillium, wild ginger, and azaleas blooming. Sempervirens Falls cascades by fallen redwoods into a crystal-clear pool. Round-trip the hike is about 4 miles, although you can cut a mile or two off if you pick up the trail from Wastahi or Huckleberry campground.

The 12-mile hike for which everybody comes to Big Basin is down to Berry Creek Falls. You start out at Park Headquarters and hike through the redwoods, up over the ridge, and down 4 miles to magnificent Berry Creek Falls, with a 70-foot drop to a clear pool and more cascades fringed with ferns. I saw these falls first after a rainstorm in the sudden light of the sun—so beautiful, I thought, Great Spirit, why are you speaking to unworthy me, with my day pack full of bologna sandwiches and a plastic baggie of dill pickles?

To get back, hike on up the staircase past Cascade Falls, Silver Falls, and Golden Falls, and follow Sunset Trail back to Park Headquarters.

Big Basin is home to black-tailed deer, raccoons, skunks, and squirrels. Rangers put up notices about mountain lions, but nobody ever sees the big cats. Even the Native Americans called them "ghosts." As rare as mountain lions are the marbled murrelets. These robin-sized seabirds hunt fish in the ocean. Nobody had ever seen them nest until, in 1974, somebody discovered a murrelet nest made of live moss up in a Big Basin redwood. In bird-watching circles, a murrelet sighting is a great coup.

The nearest supplies are in Boulder Creek, but you want to go down to Santa Cruz and at least hike along the old half-mile boardwalk. Kids will want to ride the chilling Typhoon, the horrific Hurricane, or the terror-inspiring Wave Jammer. Adults may prefer the Giant Dipper roller coaster (circa 1924) that comes from a more genteel era. There are serious beaches here in Santa Cruz, great bookstores, a major university

KEY INFORMATION

ADDRESS:	Big Basin Redwoods State Park 21600 Big Basin Hwy. Boulder Creek, CA 95006
OPERATED BY:	California State Parks
INFORMATION:	(831) 338-8860; www.bigbasin.org
OPEN:	Year-round; some closed in winter
SITES:	146 total: 69 car-camping sites, 38 walk-in sites, 31 RV sites, 8 wheelchair-accessible sites, 35 tent cabins
EACH SITE HAS:	Picnic table, fireplace
ASSIGNMENT:	By ranger
REGISTRATION:	By entrance; reserve by phone, (800) 444-7275, or online, www.reserve america.com; tent-cabin reservations, (800) 874-8368
FACILITIES:	Water, toilets, showers, wood for sale
PARKING:	At individual site
FEE:	$25; $7.50 non-refundable reservation fee
ELEVATION:	1,000 feet
RESTRICTIONS:	*Pets:* Dogs on leash only, in campground *Fires:* In fireplace *Alcohol:* No restrictions *Vehicles:* RVs up to 30 feet, trailers up to 27 feet *Other:* 14-day stay limit (7 in summer), 30 days annually; 8 people per site; reservations recommended on holidays and summer weekends

MAP

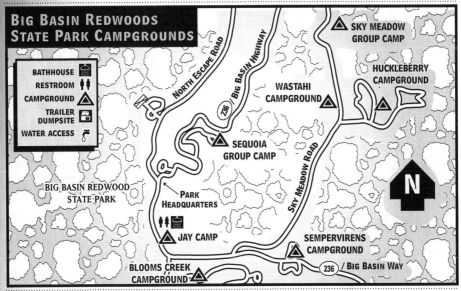

BIG BASIN REDWOODS STATE PARK CAMPGROUNDS

BATHHOUSE
RESTROOM
CAMPGROUND
TRAILER DUMPSITE
WATER ACCESS

SKY MEADOW GROUP CAMP

HUCKLEBERRY CAMPGROUND

WASTAHI CAMPGROUND

NORTH ESCAPE ROAD

BIG BASIN HIGHWAY

236

SEQUOIA GROUP CAMP

SKY MEADOW ROAD

BIG BASIN REDWOOD STATE PARK

PARK HEADQUARTERS

JAY CAMP

SEMPERVIRENS CAMPGROUND

BLOOMS CREEK CAMPGROUND

236 / BIG BASIN WAY

N

GETTING THERE

From Santa Cruz, go north on CA 9 for 12 miles to Boulder Creek. Turn left on CA 236 and drive 9 miles to the Big Basin Redwoods State Park entrance.

(even if the school mascot is the banana slug), two brew pubs, and some good places to chow down—like Aldo's at the west end of the yacht harbor.

Before you leave Big Basin, check out the 35 tent cabins on a loop road at Huckleberry Camp. Each has two full-sized beds and a wood stove, and they rent for $50 per night. Next time you need a weekend off and don't want to mount a camping trip, these babies are the answer. Bring your own sleeping bags and pillows, and wood for the stove if the season's chilly.

GPS COORDINATES

UTM Zone (WGS84) 10S

Easting 0569126

Northing 4113872

Latitude N 37° 10' 7.3560"

Longtitude W 122° 13' 16.9573"

03
BULLFROG POND
CAMPGROUND

THE TRIP TO **B**ULLFROG **P**OND feels a bit like a fairytale journey: you start in Armstrong Redwoods State Reserve in a quiet, dark redwood canyon and climb steeply into Austin Creek State Recreation Area on a tiny road, traveling through oaks and grassland to a high ridge with sweeping views and a campground sheltered by trees around a small pond. Although the campground is open all year, winter camping is soggy, and summers are sweltering. Spring is best, and autumn is fine as well, although late in the year when there's high fire danger, campfires can be prohibited.

Campsites 1 through 20 are well sheltered by evergreens, with redwoods dominating the landscape but without many understory shrubs to screen views between sites. Sites 10, 11, and 12 are close together and make a perfect spot for three families to camp together. Site 21, at a bend in the campground road, has no immediate neighbors but is small. This site is adjacent to a path connecting to Austin Creek Trail. Sites 22 and 23 sit out in the open on the shore of Bullfrog Pond, a small man-made pond where fishing for black bass is allowed (state permit required). On summer weekends, locals head to the pond in a steady stream, so these sites are not the best choice if you're seeking privacy. Site 24 is widely thought to be Austin Creek's best campsite and is usually the first claimed. Surrounded by madrone, redwood, California bay, coast live oak, and young Douglas fir, the spacious site is a 150-yard walk from the toilets and parking area.

Even though it's just a few miles from Guerneville, Bullfrog Pond Campground is a quiet destination with an abundant wildlife population. On the drive in, a bobcat ran across the road in front of us, and a flock of wild turkeys waddled up a hillside in the campground—you'll likely hear (and see) turkeys wherever

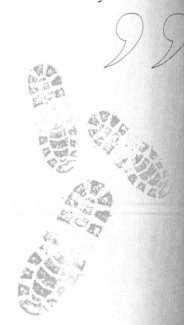

An enclave of wilderness in the midst of Sonoma County's wine country.

RATINGS

Beauty: ✿ ✿ ✿
Privacy: ✿ ✿
Spaciousness: ✿ ✿ ✿
Quiet: ✿ ✿ ✿
Security: ✿ ✿
Cleanliness: ✿ ✿ ✿

KEY INFORMATION

ADDRESS:	Bullfrog Pond Campground Austin Creek State Recreation Area 17000 Armstrong Woods Road Guerneville, CA 95446
OPERATED BY:	California State Parks
INFORMATION:	(707) 869-2015; www.parks.ca.gov
OPEN:	Year-round
SITES:	24 sites for tents only
EACH SITE HAS:	Fire ring, picnic table, food locker
ASSIGNMENT:	First come, first served; no reservations
REGISTRATION:	At Armstrong Redwoods entrance kiosk, or at the self-registration station
FACILITIES:	Drinking water, flush toilets, firewood
PARKING:	1 vehicle per site—additional parking available
FEE:	$15 per night, $6 each additional vehicle
ELEVATION:	1,200 feet
RESTRICTIONS:	*Pets:* Dogs on leash only, in campground *Fires:* In established pits/rings only; may be prohibited during high fire danger *Vehicles:* No vehicles over 20 feet long *Other:* Austin Creek also has 3 backcountry campsites, reached by a 3-mile hike—permits required.

you go at Austin Creek. At our campsite we saw a jackrabbit and heard deer walking through the woods at night. Quacking ducks on Bullfrog Pond may rouse you from your sleeping bag in the morning. Be sure to keep your food in the storage boxes or in a secure container, for marauding raccoons are bold. Wild pigs are common and are sometimes spotted in the campground, but you are more likely to encounter them on the trails. Their eyesight is poor, and there are two main pig-encounter strategies—either make a lot of noise and wave your arms, scaring them away, or quietly creep away from them, hoping to avoid their attention. These animals are not known to be aggressive, but don't provoke them—they can run faster than you and many wield tusks.

The trails at Austin Creek are steeper and tougher than those at adjacent Armstrong Redwoods. If you want an easy stroll, drive back down that steep road to the main redwood grove at Armstrong Redwoods, and walk among the giants. The Discovery Trail was designed for the visually impaired; try closing your eyes and using your other senses on the path. From the campground you can hike down into Armstrong Redwoods via East Ridge Trail and return uphill on Pool Ridge Trail, a more-than-6-mile trek that alternates between woods and grassland.

On our latest visit, we made a 4-mile loop out of Austin Creek and Gilliam Creek trails. From the campground, pick up a connecting path near site 21, and when you reach an unsigned T, turn right, then drop down to Austin Creek Trail (a fire road) and turn right (or begin from the day-use parking area across from the registration station and walk a short distance down the park road to the gated trailhead). Descend through grassland dotted with oaks, where wild-pig damage along the trail is obvious and severe. The downhill grade is relentless, but after dropping about 1,000 feet from the trailhead, Austin Creek Trail nears Gilliam Creek and levels out a bit. Look for hound's tongue and milkmaids blooming beneath black oak, California bay, and maple in March. At about the 1.5-mile mark, there's a junction at a bridge across the creek. Backpackers heading to Tom King Trail Camp turn right

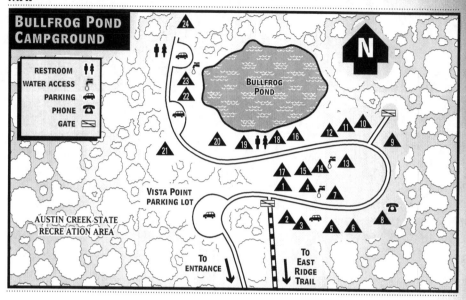

BULLFROG POND CAMPGROUND

RESTROOM	👫
WATER ACCESS	
PARKING	🚗
PHONE	☎
GATE	✉

BULLFROG POND

N

VISTA POINT
PARKING LOT

AUSTIN CREEK STATE
RECREATION AREA

TO
ENTRANCE

TO
EAST
RIDGE
TRAIL

here. In early spring we saw more than a dozen newts mating in the creek.

Follow a connecting path straight from the junction to a creek crossing (which may be impassable after heavy winter rains), then reach an undersigned junction with Gilliam Creek Trail. Turn left. It's easy going at first, as the trail weaves through the woods, keeping to a slight uphill grade. But soon Gilliam Creek Trail begins a tough climb. After a final stretch running parallel to (but obscured from) the park road, the trail ends at a small parking lot. Turn left and walk uphill on the side of the road to the junction with East Ridge Trail, and follow the trail uphill back to the campground (or simply walk on the road—it's shorter). If you have any energy left, in the late afternoon, walk up to the viewpoint adjacent to the self-registration station and watch the sun set over miles of Austin Creek's protected watershed.

Guerneville is the logical stop to fill up your car and stock up on food. You'll drive right past Korbel on the way to Austin Creek, and by the number of champagne corks in the fire pit, it looks like many campers pop in for some bubbly to be enjoyed at their campsite.

GETTING THERE

From US 101 north of Santa Rosa in Sonoma County, exit River Road. Drive west 15.5 miles on River Road into Guerneville, then turn right onto Armstrong Redwoods Road. Drive north 2.3 miles to the Armstrong Redwoods entrance kiosk and proceed 0.6 miles through the flat redwood canyon. Then, following the signs for Bullfrog Pond, continue north 2.3 miles on the one-lane narrow, winding road to the campground.

GPS COORDINATES

UTM Zone (WGS84) 10S

Easting 0499007

Northing 4268681

Latitude N 38° 33' 59.6770"

Longtitude W 123° 0' 41.0326"

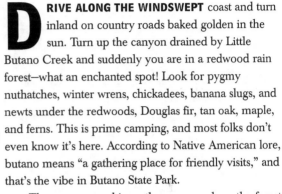

> *Quiet as a church, but with a carnival of outdoor activities around the campground.*

DRIVE ALONG THE WINDSWEPT coast and turn inland on country roads baked golden in the sun. Turn up the canyon drained by Little Butano Creek and suddenly you are in a redwood rain forest—what an enchanted spot! Look for pygmy nuthatches, winter wrens, chickadees, banana slugs, and newts under the redwoods, Douglas fir, tan oak, maple, and ferns. This is prime camping, and most folks don't even know it's here. According to Native American lore, butano means "a gathering place for friendly visits," and that's the vibe in Butano State Park.

The campground is up the canyon where the forest grows the thickest. Look for sites 22 through 39—these are the tent-only walk-in sites. At most, the walk is about 30 yards. The trees are so tall, the forest so still that camping here is like pitching a tent in a cathedral. The pitches are soft and spongy—although by fall there is a soft, red grit, so bring a drop cloth to clean your feet before entering your tent. The huge trees moderate the heat in the summer and the cold in the winter. Between the nearby rugged coast and these majestic trees, Butano State Park offers the best of two distinctly different worlds.

Hike up the Little Butano Creek Loop for a quick look at the park. The trail begins just below the campground. Cross the creek on footbridges and look for trillium, oxalis, and forget-me-not. In the spring, look for baby newts. At a junction, stay below with the creek. The paths soon come together and climb through the maples. About a mile out, either cross the creek and return to the campground via an access road, or retrace your route.

A slightly longer walk is the Jackson Flats–Six Bridges Hike. Pick up this hike down below the picnic area by the entrance booth. Head up a ridge through Douglas fir, madrone, and poison oak (don't touch).

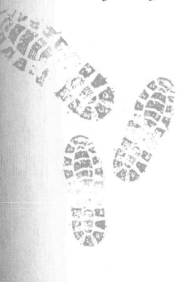

RATINGS

Beauty: ✫ ✫ ✫ ✫ ✫
Privacy: ✫ ✫ ✫
Spaciousness: ✫ ✫ ✫ ✫
Quiet: ✫ ✫ ✫ ✫ ✫
Security: ✫ ✫ ✫ ✫ ✫
Cleanliness: ✫ ✫ ✫ ✫

After a rain, look for chanterelle mushrooms (don't pick). After a mile and a half, look for a cattail marsh on your left before entering old-growth redwoods at 2 miles. This is a good place to turn around. On the way back, one option is to take the Mill Ox Trail on the left and head back to the park road—go left uphill to the campground.

To visit the beach, go left on Cloverdale Road and down Gazos Creek Road to CA 1. Go across the highway and into the Gazos Creek access parking lot. There is a pretty little beach below Gazos, Whitehouse, and Cascade canyons. Alternately, you can continue south exactly 1 mile. Park and walk over the dunes to the ocean. Now this is a great beach, with a protected cove at the south end and tidepools at the north end. A local showed me this beach and swore me to secrecy. Ha!

A little farther south find Año Nuevo State Reserve. This is truly an incredible experience. Northern elephant seals use Año Nuevo as a rookery. Spot the island and its abandoned buildings. This used to be a lighthouse facility, and folks who lived there often chased 2,000-pound elephant seals out of the kitchen garden and sometimes found them sliding down the halls of the house.

During breeding season, between December and March, male elephant seals as big as VW Beetles fight mano a mano for the ladies' favors. To see this spectacle, you have to go on a ranger-guided walk, which requires advance reservations—as early as October. Phone (800) 444-4445 for a spot. Any other time, just hiking around the reserve is wonderful. The pond is great for bird-watching—waves of different birds pass through. The beach area is pristine and protected (careful of the rips), and the visitor center has a fine exhibit in an old barn, once part of the Steele Brothers Dairy Farm.

The charming town of Pescadero is a good refueling stop—this is one of the few spots for gas near the park. Arcangeli Grocery, on Pescadero's main strip, makes incredible artichoke-studded bread and other baked delights and also stocks a small variety of grocery staples, meat, and poultry. Duarte's Tavern is a coastal institution, serving breakfast, lunch, and dinner in the

KEY INFORMATION

ADDRESS:	Butano State Park Box 3 1500 Cloverdale Road Pescadero, CA 94060
OPERATED BY:	California State Parks
INFORMATION:	(650) 879-2040; www.parks.ca.gov
OPEN:	Year-round
SITES:	39 total; 21 drive-in, 18 walk-in
EACH SITE HAS:	Picnic table, fireplace
ASSIGNMENT:	Reservations online or by phone; assigned by ranger
REGISTRATION:	By entrance; reserve by phone, (800) 444-7275, or online, www.reserve america.com
FACILITIES:	Water, flush toilets
PARKING:	At individual site
FEE:	$25; $7.50 nonrefundable reservation fee
ELEVATION:	400 feet
RESTRICTIONS:	*Pets:* Dogs on leash only, in campground and on paved park roads *Fires:* In fireplace *Alcohol:* No restrictions *Vehicles:* RVs up to 27 feet, trailers up to 24 feet *Other:* Reservations required on holidays, recommended on summer weekends; otherwise first come, first served

MAP

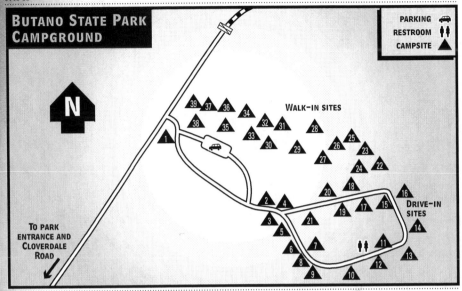

BUTANO STATE PARK CAMPGROUND

PARKING
RESTROOM
CAMPSITE

WALK-IN SITES

DRIVE-IN SITES

N

TO PARK ENTRANCE AND CLOVERDALE ROAD

GETTING THERE

From Half Moon Bay, drive 15 miles south on CA 1 to Pescadero Road on the left. Go east on Pescadero Road, past the town of Pescadero. Go right on Cloverdale Road. The park entrance is 4.5 miles on the left.

same location since 1894. The cream of artichoke soup is justly famous, but the cream of green chili is also delicious; some folks ask for a mixture of the two soups in one bowl. May through September you can pick your own strawberries and olallieberries at Phipps Country Store and Farm, on the outskirts of Pescadero. For just-off-the-boat seafood, take a scenic drive north to Pillar Point harbor in Princeton, 4 miles past Half Moon Bay. If you'd rather linger near Pescadero, buy picnic fixings and head to Bean Hollow State Beach, where you can watch the waves crash on the shoreline.

GPS COORDINATES

UTM Zone (WGS84) 10S
Easting 0557474
Northing 4119249
Latitude N 37° 13' 4.6775"
Longtitude W 122° 21' 7.9235"

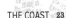

05
DILLON CREEK CAMPGROUND

ALL RANGERS WILL TELL YOU Dillon Creek Campground is a good campground. "Ah, Dillon," the rangers say and smile. "The river down there is nice." Rangers love Dillon because it is a model campground. The campground host's trailer sits right at the entrance to where the Dillon campsites file back along the hill. And, located by CA 96, Dillon is easy to patrol. I spoke to the campground host who said, "We had an unruly bear here once and I called for help on my mobile phone. The law was here in 10 minutes." Did they arrest the bear? I forgot to ask.

A steep trail leads down to Dillon Creek, where there is one great swimming hole near the campground, as well as dozens of more secluded ones upstream. Although Dillon Creek can flow ferociously in the spring flood, the current does not present the danger of the mighty Klamath that flows right across CA 89 from Dillon, where everybody goes for salmon and the famous steelhead.

Beginning in the fall, the name of the game here is steelhead. For anglers, this means the Klamath River in the winter, cold nights around a smoky campfire telling fish stories, and that one hard bite on the line that can only mean steelhead! What's a steelhead?

Steelhead are a kind of rainbow trout. Like salmon, steelhead spend some of their lives in the ocean, feeding and growing faster than their exclusively freshwater cousins, rainbow trout, then head up rivers like the Klamath to spawn. Steelhead average 10 pounds (some grow to 20 or more). Unlike salmon, steelhead do not die after spawning. They can come back two or three times to spawn again.

Steelhead and salmon look mostly alike. Steelhead have 9 to 12 bones or rays in their anal fin, and salmon have 13 to 19. (The anal fin is the bottom fin in front of the tail and behind the vent.) Steelhead have small,

> *Good steelhead fishing and a great swimming hole, right in the middle of the best river rafting!*

RATINGS

Beauty: ✿ ✿ ✿ ✿ ✿
Privacy: ✿ ✿ ✿ ✿
Spaciousness: ✿ ✿ ✿
Quiet: ✿ ✿ ✿
Security: ✿ ✿ ✿ ✿ ✿
Cleanliness: ✿ ✿ ✿ ✿

KEY INFORMATION

ADDRESS: Dillon Creek
Campground
Klamath National
Forest
Orleans Ranger
District
P.O. Drawer 410
Orleans, CA 95556

OPERATED BY: U.S. Forest Service

INFORMATION: (530) 627-3291;
www.fs.fed.us/r5/
klamath

OPEN: May–October

SITES: 10 sites for tents
only, 11 sites for
tents or RVs

EACH SITE HAS: Picnic table, fireplace, grills

ASSIGNMENT: First come, first
served;
no reservations

REGISTRATION: By entrance

FACILITIES: Water, vault toilets,
wheelchair
accessibility

PARKING: At individual site

FEE: $10 plus $5 day-use
fee; $5 additional
vehicle

ELEVATION: 800 feet

RESTRICTIONS: *Pets:* On leash only
Fires: In fireplace
Alcohol: No
restrictions
Vehicles: No trailers
over 22 feet

round, black spots on their back, and salmon have larger, irregular spots and lack the broad red stripe the steelhead get after being in freshwater for a while.

Peak months for catching big steelhead are January, February, and March. But littler ones (half-pounders) come into the Klamath in the spring and spend the summer in big river pools before spawning in the fall rains. And other little guys and some big mothers will come into the Klamath as early as August. How you fish steelhead depends on how the run is— and how your luck is. Once you hook a steelhead, it takes skill to land one, for steelhead are acrobatic, hard-fighting fish. Good luck! Of course, to decrease the odds, ask around in Happy Camp (don't you just love the name of that town?) for a good fishing guide.

Last time I was in Dillon, the fall run of steelhead had not arrived. The campground host told me anglers were catching steelhead down near Somes Bar. Only mildly disappointed, we put on our water shoes and went down to the swimming hole. It was nice and hot. We had good fun working our way up Dillon Creek River, checking things out. We took a picnic, found a nice warm rock next to a clear pool, and hung out for the afternoon.

The next day, we found a trail that ran up the north side of Dillon Creek, and followed it up a mile or so. Later I heard that this trail is used by the Fish and Game people, who hike up to where Dillon Creek forks to do a fish count. South of the campground entrance, FS 13N35 heads up the shoulder of Dillon Mountain (4,679 feet). We hiked it until it got too steep and the sun got too hot.

There is also a trail that heads up the mountain behind the campground, but I couldn't find anyone who knew where it went. Basically, by the time you get as far out in the woods as Dillon Creek Campground, folks don't spend much time marking trails. And, since this is rugged-individualist country—land of tacked-together shacks tied to the Klamath River bank with rusty cables, and pot plantations among the red-woods—it is not a healthy idea to lunge blindly off into the woods. You might end up as fertilizer. Try to stick to the river bank and to semiofficial trails or roads.

MAP

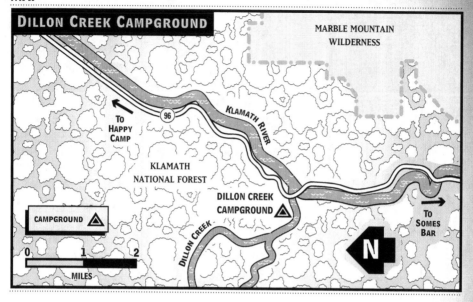

DILLON CREEK CAMPGROUND

MARBLE MOUNTAIN
WILDERNESS

To
HAPPY
CAMP

96

KLAMATH RIVER

KLAMATH
NATIONAL FOREST

DILLON CREEK
CAMPGROUND

CAMPGROUND

DILLON CREEK

To
SOMES
BAR

N

0   1   2

MILES

For adventure, try river rafting. Happy Camp is full of experienced outfits happy to take you down the river. I recommend going with an outfit your first couple of times out before trying anything hasty. Proper equipment is a must; a helmet and life jacket can make a huge difference when you, your spouse, or your kid is dumped suddenly into the rapids.

Happy Camp has a good supermarket (as well as good hamburgers at the western-style bar-cafe in town). I saw flyers up in town for folks who will take you gold panning and horseback riding. The Happy Camp Ranger Station has all the details. This little town seems friendly as well as happy.

GETTING THERE

From Somes Bar, drive 15 miles north on CA 96. Or drive 25 miles south of Happy Camp on CA 96.

GPS COORDINATES

UTM Zone (WGS84) 10T

Easting 0454659

Northing 4602552

Latitude N 41° 34' 24.1139"

Longtitude W 123° 32' 37.9031"

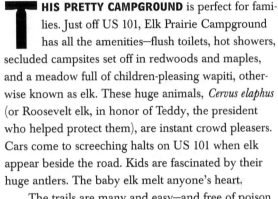

*Redwoods, the beach,
and the elk will amuse
the kids on a summer
family vacation.*

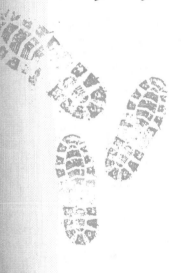

THIS PRETTY CAMPGROUND is perfect for families. Just off US 101, Elk Prairie Campground has all the amenities—flush toilets, hot showers, secluded campsites set off in redwoods and maples, and a meadow full of children-pleasing wapiti, otherwise known as elk. These huge animals, *Cervus elaphus* (or Roosevelt elk, in honor of Teddy, the president who helped protect them), are instant crowd pleasers. Cars come to screeching halts on US 101 when elk appear beside the road. Kids are fascinated by their huge antlers. The baby elk melt anyone's heart.

The trails are many and easy—and free of poison oak! A few miles away (by car or foot) is the most beautiful, most secluded sandy beach in all of California. Orick, a few miles to the south, has all the redwood burls the world could ever desire, groceries, and brunches at Rolf's Park Cafe—a German schnitzel house featuring elk steak.

The absolute best time to come is in September and October when the sun shines. Summer is warmer, but expect some fog and be prepared to dress for it. Spring has rainy spells but also wildflowers.

Winter is a bear, and unless you arrive between huge storms, prepare to be wet—although some folks love it this way. Seal the seams on your tent. The way it rains up here, water will come up through untreated seams to make a lap pool on the floor of your tent. Bring a garden trowel to ditch around the tent and a good drop cloth to lay under the tent. Fold the sides of the drop cloth up under the tent, so the water won't pool between the tent floor and the drop cloth. Also, bring good books and playing cards.

The elk don't mind the wet. They're just glad not to be hunted to near extermination for their meat, hide, and upper canine teeth. Once these elk ranged over most of the continent—from the Berkshires in

RATINGS

Beauty: ✪ ✪ ✪ ✪ ✪
Privacy: ✪ ✪ ✪ ✪ ✪
Spaciousness: ✪ ✪ ✪
Quiet: ✪ ✪ ✪
Security: ✪ ✪ ✪ ✪ ✪
Cleanliness: ✪ ✪ ✪ ✪ ✪

western Massachusetts to southern New Mexico. By 1912, the elk herd was down to about 15 elk. They made their last stand here in Prairie Creek Redwoods State Park.

Elk love elk. Very gregarious, elk band together even at the risk of running out of pasture. Known for their huge, intimidating antlers, bull elk are paper tigers. The antlers seem to be mostly show. When elk fight, they strike with their front feet and use the antlers for a chopping, downward motion. Most important for the bull elk is his bugle—the low note rising a full octave to a sweet, mellow crescendo, dropping by degrees to the first note, then a few coughing grunts. The elk bulls here are big bark and little bite. Of course, humanoids should not approach elk or get in their way.

Listen to AM radio 1610 while in the park. This is elk local news and will tell you where the herd is. A good elk-spotting hike is around Elk Prairie. Bring binoculars. A little more than 2 miles, the loop should take a little over an hour. Start near campsite 67 and follow the trail south through Sitka spruce and alder. Cross a little stream, then head into the open prairie. At a break in the fence, head across the prairie to the parkway, cross it, and pick up the trail on the other side. This trail will parallel the parkway. Look for signs of elk—tracks, bark rubbed off, tender shoots eaten, elk wallows—and the elk herd itself. Keep going until you reach a junction with the Rhododendron and Cathedral Trees trails. Go left and circle back to the campground, going under the parkway by the kiosk and visitor center.

Another good hike is down to Fern Canyon and the beach via the James Irvine Trail. This is a day hike, about 8 miles round-trip, so take water and food. To pick up the James Irvine Trail, take the nature trail by the visitor center, cross Prairie Creek on a bridge, and continue past the start of the Prairie Creek Trail until you see the James Irvine Trail. The trail follows Godwood Creek through virgin redwood, Sitka spruce, Douglas fir, and hemlock. At almost 3 miles you'll cross a bridge over the headwater of Home Creek. Follow Home Creek down into Fern Canyon. Gold Bluffs Beach is just beyond. Lots of folks drive through the park to visit Fern Canyon.

KEY INFORMATION

ADDRESS:	Elk Prairie Campground Prairie Creek Redwoods State Park 127077 Newton B. Drury Parkway Orick, CA 95555
OPERATED BY:	California State Parks
INFORMATION:	(707) 464-6101, ext. 5301; www.parks.ca.gov
OPEN:	Year-round
SITES:	76 sites for tents or RVs; 3 wheelchair-accessible sites
EACH SITE HAS:	Picnic table, fire ring
ASSIGNMENT:	Reservation recommended May–September; otherwise first come, first served
REGISTRATION:	By entrance; reserve by phone, (800) 444-7275, or online, www.reserve america.com
FACILITIES:	Water, flush toilets, showers, wood for sale
PARKING:	At individual site
FEE:	$20; $7.50 non-refundable reservation fee
ELEVATION:	150 feet
RESTRICTIONS:	*Pets:* On leash only *Fires:* In fire ring *Alcohol:* No restrictions *Vehicles:* RVs up to 27 feet, trailers up to 24 feet

MAP

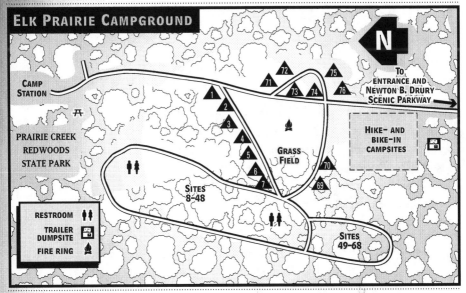

ELK PRAIRIE CAMPGROUND

N

CAMP
STATION

PRAIRIE CREEK
REDWOODS
STATE PARK

72
71
75
73 74
76

To
ENTRANCE AND
NEWTON B. DRURY
SCENIC PARKWAY

HIKE- AND
BIKE-IN
CAMPSITES

1
2
3
4
5
6
7

GRASS
FIELD

70
69

SITES
8-48

RESTROOM
TRAILER
DUMPSITE
FIRE RING

SITES
49-68

GETTING THERE

From Orick, drive 6 miles
north on US 101. Go left on
the Newton B. Drury Scenic
Parkway, and left again into
Elk Prairie Campground.

Look out for the famous banana slug, bright yellow and about six inches long. They crawl around conspicuously and like to eat all sorts of forest litter and debris. So famous indeed, the slug has been proposed as the California state mollusk. They are hermaphrodites and have penises as long as their bodies. When they mate, they impregnate each other, thus neatly opting out of the war between the sexes. Camp in August and attend the official Banana Slug Derby!

GPS COORDINATES

UTM Zone (WGS84) 10T

Easting 0414714

Northing 4584448

Latitude N 41° 24' 25.3981"

Longtitude W 124° 1' 13.3681"

GOLD BLUFFS BEACH HAS TO BE the prettiest sand beach in California. Steep sandstone cliffs rise up to more eroded cliffs spiked with towering Sitka spruce. The salt-and-pepper sand beach stretches as far as the eye can see in both directions. There's a sea mist kicked up by the surf that bathes the scene with billowing white. The waves break far out and slowly comb to shore. What an incredible beach!

And the Gold Bluffs Beach Campground is the best beach campground on the California coast. There are 25 sites, available on a first-come, first-served basis, all in the dunes 100 yards back from the beach. Some sites have railroad-tie wind shelters. Behind you are the wildflowered bluffs, ahead a couple thousand miles of blue water—and Hawaii. Surf-fish for perch, and dip for smelt at night.

Wind scours the sand. The beach and the campground are always clean, by morning pristine—the footprints and debris of the day before blown away in the night. The facilities are also clean, and the solar showers are hot if the sun shines. The beach is nice and level, perfect for hiking and beach combing. The mist keeps the sun from being too hot, and that sea breeze always blows sweet in your face. Nothing could be more perfect—except for the weather.

Don't expect great weather on Gold Bluffs Beach unless you come in September or October, which are the premium weather months in this part of the world. From October to April, Gold Bluffs Beach gets a ton of rain. Of course, rain here is cosmic symphonics—the clouds billow, blacken, and boil across the sky; the wind brings rain slashing sideways into the sand; and the surf churns up gray to reflect the sky. Suddenly you know why your tent is double-stitched and thank the Lord you remembered to seal your seams against the wet. It rains. Just south of here, the Lost Coast can get

> *The prettiest, most remote beach camping in California.*

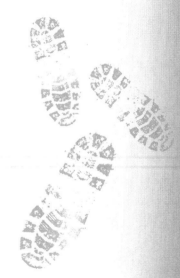

RATINGS

Beauty: ✩ ✩ ✩ ✩ ✩
Privacy: ✩ ✩ ✩
Spaciousness: ✩ ✩ ✩
Quiet: ✩ ✩ ✩ ✩ ✩
Security: ✩ ✩ ✩ ✩ ✩
Cleanliness: ✩ ✩ ✩ ✩ ✩

KEY INFORMATION

ADDRESS: Gold Bluffs Beach Campground Prairie Creek Redwoods State Park 127077 Newton B. Drury Parkway Orick, CA 95555

OPERATED BY: California State Parks

INFORMATION: (707) 464-6101, ext. 5301; www.parks.ca.gov

OPEN: Year-round

SITES: 25 sites for tents or small RVs

EACH SITE HAS: Picnic table, fireplace, bear box

ASSIGNMENT: Reservations recommended May–September; otherwise first come, first served

REGISTRATION: By entrance; reserve by phone, (800) 444-7275, or online, www.reserve america.com

FACILITIES: Water, flush toilets, solar showers

PARKING: At individual site

FEE: $20; $7.50 non-refundable reservation fee

ELEVATION: 10 feet

RESTRICTIONS: *Pets:* On leash only
Fires: In fireplace
Alcohol: No restrictions
Vehicles: RVs up to 20 feet, no trailers
Other: Store food in bear boxes; canoeing requires a permit

up to 200 inches of rain yearly. Think about it. That's 16 feet of water—10 feet over the average guy's head!

April and May are windy with some rainstorms, and the wildflowers start growing like crazy on the bluffs. Look for Indian paintbrush, cow parsnip, iris, and lupine. In June, July, and August expect hot, sunny summer days alternating with thick fog. But September and October are heaven, when the beach is at its most beautiful, the bluffs are cooked gold, and the sea is a deep green.

There is no cover at the campground, so think about how to manage the sun and wind. Bring big hats and lots of sunblock, and try to improvise shade. With rope and a sturdy tarp, you can usually arrange a makeshift sun shelter. Kelty sells a sunshade for about $150 that looks like a grounded kite. We used it once, and it held up agreeably to less-than-hurricane winds, when most other dining canopies would have blown halfway to Kansas. I think the most portable arrangement is a sombrero and a cheap sun umbrella that clamps on to your aluminum chair (umbrellas can be found next to the aluminum chairs in your favorite discount store).

The first folks here were the Yurok Indians, who didn't have these amenities. They lived in a village by the lagoon, just south of where Davison Road hits the beach. Then came the gold miners in 1850, who found flecks of gold mixed with the gray-and-black sand at Gold Bluffs Beach. Miners flooded the area and were terribly disappointed when they discovered that the gold was bound so tightly to the sand that it had to be extracted with quicksilver sluice boxes. And the gold-bearing sand was only available when waves crashed against the bluff and dislodged big chunks of the bank. Most of the miners fled for other diggin's.

A few stayed and used mules to carry the sand ore up to the bluffs. Apparently, the mule trips were timed so the animals could avoid the waves and reach their destination dry. In those days, the beach was much narrower than now. As the beach widened, the waves stopped cutting away at the bluff, and all mining stopped. Still, look above Carruther's Cove for the flume that cuts across the hillside. On the knoll above

MAP

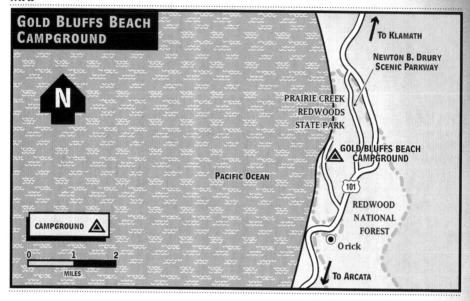

GOLD BLUFFS BEACH CAMPGROUND

To Klamath

Newton B. Drury Scenic Parkway

Prairie Creek Redwoods State Park

Gold Bluffs Beach Campground

Pacific Ocean

101

Redwood National Forest

Orick

To Arcata

CAMPGROUND

0   1   2

MILES

N

Major Creek there are still some boards left from Chapman's Union Gold Bluff Mine.

Hiking here is on the beach and on the trails heading east to Elk Prairie Campground. The short loop around Fern Canyon is a don't-miss jaunt. With 50-foot walls of ferns, Fern Canyon sits a couple miles north of Gold Bluffs Beach Campground. The most common fern here is the five-finger fern, a relative of the maidenhair fern. The Yuroks gathered these ferns for the black stems they wove into their incredible baskets. Look for the banana slug and the omnivorous Pacific giant salamander. Also, look for winter wrens, the water ouzel, and the great blue heron.

GETTING THERE

From Orick, go 3 miles north on US 101 to Davison Road on the left. Go 4 miles on Davison Road to Gold Bluffs Beach Campground. Drive carefully; the road is narrow, unpaved, and slippery when wet.

GPS COORDINATES

UTM Zone (WGS84) 10T

Easting 0414009

Northing 4577992

Latitude N 41° 20' 55.8094"

Longtitude W 124° 1' 40.4326"

08
JEDEDIAH SMITH REDWOODS STATE PARK CAMPGROUND

> *The most northern of California's beautiful Redwoods State Parks— and the sun shines through the summer fog!*

BY THE TIME THE ROAD-WEARY camper arrives at Jedediah Smith Redwoods State Park near the Oregon border, he's bound to throw up his hands and plead, "Oh, Lord, not another beautiful Redwoods State Park!"

Jedediah Smith Redwoods State Park is gorgeous. Not only does the Smith River run by the campground for unparalleled fishing, canoeing, kayaking, and swimming, but the hiking is also great. The wild Smith River National Recreation Area is next door, and the summer weather is usually nice and sunny. Jedediah Smith Campground is fortuitously far enough east to escape the cool summer fog that plagues other state parks in redwood country. Hallelujah! The kids can paddle happily around in the river (old sneakers or water shoes of some sort are a must) while Dad sits in his lawn chair by the river and casts for trout. Meanwhile, the rays of sun will stream through the crowns of the high redwoods and splash on the ground.

Jedediah Smith Campground should really be named Sitragitum or Tcunsultum Campground for either of the two Tolowa Native American villages that were in the area, because namesake Jedediah Smith was here only less than a day in 1828 on his way to getting most of his men rubbed out in Oregon. The famous Bible-toting pathfinder, Smith, made the mistake of humiliating an Umpqua tribesman whom they suspected of stealing an ax. Big mistake. Two days later, a hundred Umpqua warriors attacked and killed 16 of Smith's long-haired and buckskin-fringed trappers. Only two trappers fought their way to safety. Smith just happened to be off scouting when the attack happened, and he learned the news from one of the survivors. Smith explored on—finally losing his hair a few years later to some Comanche by a water hole on the Arkansas River.

RATINGS

Beauty: ✿ ✿ ✿ ✿ ✿
Privacy: ✿ ✿ ✿
Spaciousness: ✿ ✿ ✿
Quiet: ✿ ✿ ✿
Security: ✿ ✿ ✿ ✿ ✿
Cleanliness: ✿ ✿ ✿ ✿

Most of the good hiking from Jedediah Smith Campground is across the Smith River. During the summer, there is a footbridge across the river to connect with the Hiouchi Trail. The footbridge is by the winter boat launch between campsites 84 and 86. The rest of the year prepare to get your feet wet. Remember, it's hard walking on all that river rock in your bare feet, so bring some water shoes. After crossing the summer bridge, or wading the river, go left for the Mill Creek Trail. The trail follows Mill Creek southeast to Howland Road and the Boy Scout Tree Road. Go right for the Simpson–Reed Discovery Trail and the Hatton Loop, which are must-see excursions. (To access them by car, just exit the Jedediah Smith Campground and drive 2 miles west on US 199.)

Across the highway from the Hatton Loop, the Simpson-Reed Discovery Trail is wonderfully done. Taking only about half an hour to make the loop, I learned all kinds of things about the coastal redwoods and the plants that live around them—like how to identify the redwood sorrel with its purple undersides and pink flowers, and why hemlock stands on its roots. Called the octopus tree, hemlock has seeds that germinate on decaying redwood logs. Their roots straddle redwood logs, which finally rot totally away, leaving the hemlock roots looking like wooden legs. I also learned that the huge redwoods come from tiny seeds—a pound of redwood seeds would start a hundred thousand trees.

If you tire of the bustle of Jedediah Smith Campground, head down to Big Flat Campground off South Fork Road for some real peace and quiet. Big Flat is in the Smith River National Recreation Area, an amazing 305,337-acre hunk of wilderness in the Six River National Forest. The campground has 28 sites but no potable water. Sites cost $8 per night. To reach Big Flat Campground, just turn south on South Fork Road. Turn left after crossing the second bridge, and travel 12 miles on South Fork Road to French Hill Road. Turn left on French Hill Road and go 100 feet to the Big Flat Campground entrance on the left.

The drive south on South Fork Road is sublime. The Smith River, the last wild, undammed river in

KEY INFORMATION

ADDRESS:	Jedediah Smith Redwoods State Park 1111 Second Street Crescent City, CA 95531
OPERATED BY:	California State Parks
INFORMATION:	(707) 458-3018, (707) 458-3496; www.parks.ca.gov
OPEN:	Year-round
SITES:	86 sites for tents or RVs
EACH SITE HAS:	Picnic table, fireplace, cupboard
ASSIGNMENT:	First come, first served; reservations recommended
REGISTRATION:	By entrance; reserve by phone, (800) 444-7275, or online, www.reserve america.com
FACILITIES:	Water, flush toilets, showers, wood for sale, wheelchair-accessible sites
PARKING:	At individual site
FEE:	$20; $7.50 non-refundable reservation fee
ELEVATION:	150 feet
RESTRICTIONS:	*Pets:* Leashed dogs allowed in campground, not on trails *Fires:* In fireplace *Alcohol:* No restrictions *Vehicles:* RVs and trailers up to 35 feet *Other:* Reservations recommended on holidays and summer weekends; 15-day stay limit (3 days for hike and bike sites)

MAP

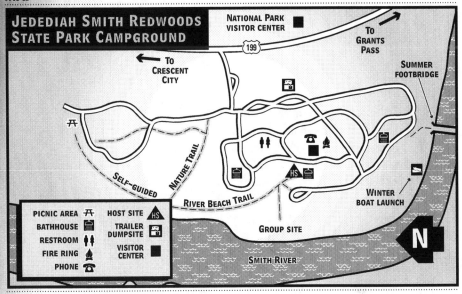

From Crescent City, go 9 miles east on US 199. The Jedediah Smith Campground is on your right before you get to Hiouchi.

California, runs through granite gorges, through rapids, down into deep pools. All along the road there are parking spots where you can leave the car and hike down to the river. (This is fine bicycling!) Most of the trails from the parking spots head for the best steelhead bank fishing.

The nearest supply from Jedediah Smith Campground is Hiouchi, a few hundred yards east. Hiouchi has a gas station, a small market, a cafe, and a decent RV park with a grass field to camp on if Jedediah Smith is packed in.

If you tire of camp grub, head down to Crescent City to the Harbor View Grotto restaurant on Citizen's Dock Road, or try the Ship Ashore restaurant up in Smith River, just off US 101. Eat great seafood and look out over the Smith River estuary. Life can't get any better.

GPS COORDINATES

UTM Zone (WGS84) 10T

Easting 0410126

Northing 4628820

Latitude N 41° 48' 22.1617

Longtitude W 124° 4' 54.9082

09
LETTS LAKE
CAMPGROUND

WITH FOUR CAMPGROUND LOOPS Letts Lake may at first sound gargantuan. But as it turns out, with only 42 sites total, Letts Lake is rather small. And quiet. It is hard to say why, but even when the campground is more than half full, Letts Lake is very peaceful. During the night, frogs croak around the lake and the wind whispers softly through the pines, and during the day, since motorized vehicles are not permitted on the lake, sounds of the soft splashes of paddles and the whirr of fishing reels barely interrupt the peaceful scene.

In summer, when heat bakes the Central Valley, campers flock to the mountains for some thermal relief, and Letts Lake fills quickly. In early spring and in autumn when the kids go back to school, the place is pretty serene. The main campground loop, closest to the entrance and right on the lake, has 18 sites and is open all year. Yes, it does snow here, so you have to make your way via unplowed roads, but the campground is open in winter.

At the main campground, sites are arranged in a small, shallow, bowl-like valley surrounded by low forested ridges. Ponderosa pine, young sugar pine, and black oak provide almost complete shade but little privacy. Two sites sit directly on the shoreline. The three other campground loops open in mid-May and are slightly uphill from the lake. These three loops are small, with sites six to ten, thanks to copious amounts of manzanita accompanying more pines and black oak. The second loop (Saddle), with sites offering partially screened views of the lake, may be our favorite. If you are new to the complex, stop at the camp host site, near the campground entrance, and ask for a site suggestion.

Wake up at Letts Lake when the sun creeps over the ridge and spills light into the campground, then

> *Small, charming campgrounds make a wonderful escape from sweltering summer temperatures.*

RATINGS

Beauty: ✩ ✩ ✩ ✩
Site Privacy: ✩ ✩ ✩
Spaciousness: ✩ ✩ ✩ ✩
Quiet: ✩ ✩ ✩ ✩
Security: ✩ ✩ ✩
Cleanliness: ✩ ✩ ✩ ✩ ✩

ADDRESS: Letts Lake Campground Mendocino National Forest 5171 Elk Creek–Stonyford Road P.O. Box 160 Stonyford, CA 95979

OPERATED BY: Mendocino National Forest

INFORMATION: (530) 963-3128; www.fs.fed.us/r5/mendocino/recreation

OPEN: 4 sections: 1 loop is open year-round unless snow closes road; remaining 3 loops are open May 15–October 15

SITES: 44 sites for tents and RVs

EACH SITE HAS: Fire ring, picnic table

ASSIGNMENT: First come, first served no reservations

REGISTRATION: Self register at entrance

FACILITIES: Drinking water, vault toilets, handicapped-accessible sites

PARKING: At individual site

FEE: $12

ELEVATION: 4,500 feet

RESTRICTIONS: *Pets:* Must be kept on leash at all times *Fires:* In established pits/rings only *Alcohol:* No restrictions *Alcohol:* No restrictions *Other:* 14-day stay limit *Vehicles:* 2 per site; RVs up to 20 feet

spend the day fishing for rainbow trout (no live bait permitted) or canoeing the placid waters. If you don't care to fish, swim, paddle, or canoe, you can walk the 1.25 miles around the lake to stretch your legs. Want a hike? Jump in your car and drive to the Snow Mountain trailhead, return to M10 (the main roads in Mendocino National Forest are designated with the letter M and a number) and turn left, then drive west (still dirt) on M10 to the spur marked to Summit Springs. The hike to the top of Snow Mountain is an 8-mile round-trip through woods and exposed hillsides, with moderate elevation gain. Expect excellent views at the top.

Letts Lake is a drowned valley with a bloody history. Brothers Jack and David Lett left Tennessee and settled in this remote area in 1855, where they made a life for themselves ranching. In 1877, the brothers attempted to run off a man who was squatting on their land, and guns were drawn; Jack and David Lett were killed. Today, a historical plaque marks the spot of the confrontation, at the edge of the boat launch. The lake was built in the early 1950s.

Stonyford is a small, sleepy sort of town, with limited provisions available. There is one gas station, a few shops, and the Stonyford Work Station, where you can ask about current road and campground conditions.

The main roads in the forest are quite rugged, sometimes rocky, but well maintained and perfectly passable for most passenger cars. If you drive a high-clearance vehicle and elect to roam around the Mendocino National Forest, come prepared. Make sure you carry emergency supplies, plenty of gas, and a detailed map. Check road conditions with the ranger station at Stonyford, particularly if you plan on crossing west through the forest to Lake Pillsbury or Upper Lake. In summer the roads are dry and stable, but as late as May some of the secondary roads (the ones with the strings of letters and numbers) may be muddy and even feature water crossings; also, it's not uncommon for some roads (even major ones) to be closed due to severe landslide and storm damage.

On the way to Letts Lake the route takes you past several other summer camping options, most of which are closed in winter. The campgrounds right off the

MAP

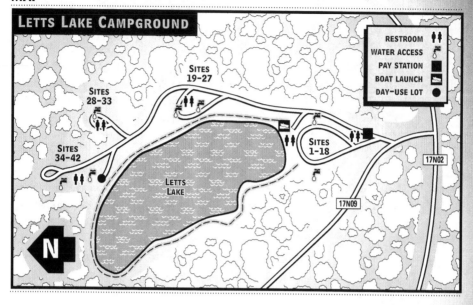

LETTS LAKE CAMPGROUND

SITES
19–27

SITES
28–33

SITES
34–42

SITES
1–18

LETTS
LAKE

RESTROOM
WATER ACCESS
PAY STATION
BOAT LAUNCH
DAY–USE LOT

17N02

17N09

N

road near Fouts Springs are primarily base camps for OHV (off-highway vehicle) riding. Dixie Glade is next, a small campground that provides direct trail access to Snow Mountain Wilderness. Mill Valley campground, with 15 sites at Lily Pond, is another option: this is the last campground before Letts Lake. If you want to push farther into the wilderness, continue past Letts Lake on FS 17N02 to MR5, then follow M5 south to Cedar Camp, near Goat Mountain, a campground with just 5 sites.

GPS COORDINATES

UTM Zone (WGS84) 10S

Easting 0525107

Northing 4350413

Latitude N 39° 18' 9.8566"

Longtitude W 122° 42' 31.7125"

GETTING THERE

From I-5 in Colusa County, exit Maxwell Road. Turn west and drive 9.5 miles to a T-junction with Sites–Stonyford Road. Turn right. Drive 13.7 miles to a junction with Lodaga–Stonyford Road; turn right. Continue 6.5 miles to Stonyford, then turn left onto Market Street. Turn left onto Fouts Springs Road (M10). After 12 miles, the paved road turns to dirt. Go another 1.6 miles, then bear left onto FS 17N02. After 3 miles, turn right at the sign for Letts Lake onto FS 17N09, then proceed to the campground entrance.

10
MACKERRICHER
STATE PARK
CAMPGROUNDS

> *MacKerricher State Park has everything but the promise of sunny weather.*

WHAT CAMPGROUND SITS NEAR 8 miles of beach, a beautiful headland, rolling dunes, lowland forest, a freshwater lake, and hundreds of snoozing harbor seals? MacKerricher State Park Campground is cheek to jowl with all of the above.

The park offers hiking, cycling, surfing, canoeing, fishing, and horseback riding. Thank Canadian-born dairy farmer Duncan MacKerricher, who bought the land for $1.25 an acre back in 1868 and whose family later deeded it to the great state of California, specifying that access to the land be free in perpetuity.

The four campground loops—East Pinewood, West Pinewood, Cleone, and Surfwood—are pretty close together. East Pinewood is closer to the road. Cleone is a little closer to Cleone Pond. Surfwood is down by the beach but near the main beach traffic. I like West Pinewood best, because it is off the highway and near the Haul Road Trail and an uncrowded beach. All the sites in all the loops are wonderfully separated and private. This is a first-class campground. There are even ten walk-in campsites (less than 50 yards away) in the Surfwood Loop for even more privacy. What a great park!

Even though the campsites are protected by pines, brush, and ferns, come prepared for wind and rain. Weather on the Mendocino coast is unpredictable, though the scenery is often most beautiful when the weather is inclement. Sometimes, of course, the sun will shine for months.

Cleone Pond is perfect for launching a canoe or kayak, and good too for trout when stocked and for some big, wary bass. The fishing here is relaxing, with the crash of the ocean waves only a sand dune away. There's a good mile walk around the pond through marsh, cattail, and bishop pine.

Take the Seal Point Trail and hike a few hundred

RATINGS

Beauty: ✿ ✿ ✿ ✿ ✿
Privacy: ✿ ✿ ✿ ✿ ✿
Spaciousness: ✿ ✿ ✿ ✿
Quiet: ✿ ✿ ✿
Security: ✿ ✿ ✿ ✿ ✿
Cleanliness: ✿ ✿ ✿ ✿

yards out on the walkway to Seal Rocks, where you should see tons of seals sleeping like sleek duffel bags on the rocks. Remember to bring binoculars to discern their cute little whiskered faces. Check out all the pretty spots on their creamy-to-dark-brown bodies. These critters spend most of their time copping Z's, but they will all dive into the water at the sign of danger (an alarm bark). They can dive to 300 feet and stay submerged up to 28 minutes. Feeding time is when the tide comes in. Sometimes they head up the rivers with the tide to eat, then haul out at low tide and snooze some more.

There is pretty good rock fishing north of Seal Rocks. Locals use squid for bait and tobacco-sack weights. The fishing stores sell these little fabric tobacco sacks for next to nothing; you can fill them with sand or small rocks and tie on to your line as weight. When the weight tangles up in the rocks, just give a pull and the tobacco sack weight breaks off, leaving you with your rock fish on the hook. Watch for rogue waves—the sudden big ones that come out of nowhere and threaten to suck you out to China.

It's fun, too, to go tidepooling in the rocks at low tide. Or poke-poling! Here's what you do. Wear old sneakers and swimming shorts. Get a bamboo pole and attach a fishing hook on a two-inch bit of wire to the end of the pole. Bait the hook with squid or mussels (rumors fly about the efficacy of abalone). Go around the tidepools in the shallow reef areas (best in minus tides) and stick the bait down under every rock and crevice. You'll get eels and rockfish and maybe small octopus. Serious poke-polers wear wetsuit bottoms so they can stay out longer. Bring a burlap sack for the booty.

Good bicycling awaits on the 7-mile Haul Road bicycle route that goes from the north side of Pudding Creek to the south, all the way north to the mouth of Ten Mile River. There's also decent cycling on the Fort Bragg Sherwood Road that heads out in Fort Bragg as Oak Avenue. Great fun for everybody is the horseback riding. Ricochet Ridge Ranch in Cleone just north of the MacKerricher State Park entrance has

KEY INFORMATION

ADDRESS: MacKerricher State Park
24100 MacKerricher Road
Fort Bragg, CA 95437

OPERATED BY: California State Parks

INFORMATION: (707) 937-5804; www.parks.ca.gov

OPEN: Year-round

SITES: 148 sites for tents or RVs; 10 walk-in sites (a 50-yard walk away); 2 group sites

EACH SITE HAS: Picnic table, fireplace, food-storage cabinet

ASSIGNMENT: First come, first served; reservations required

REGISTRATION: By entrance; reserve by phone, (800) 444-7275, or online, www.reserve america.com

FACILITIES: Water, flush toilets, hot showers, wood for sale, wheelchair-accessible sites; Wi-Fi access near visitor center

PARKING: At individual site

FEE: $25 ($20 off-season); $7.50 nonrefundable reservation fee

ELEVATION: 50 feet

RESTRICTIONS: *Pets:* On leash only
Fires: In fireplace
Alcohol: No restrictions
Vehicles: RVs and trailers up to 35 feet; 3 vehicles per campsite
Other: Reservations recommended in summer

MAP

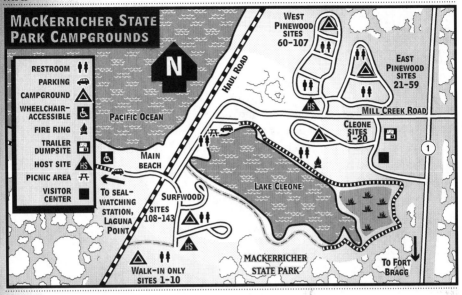

MACKERRICHER STATE PARK CAMPGROUNDS

RESTROOM
PARKING
CAMPGROUND
WHEELCHAIR-ACCESSIBLE
FIRE RING
TRAILER DUMPSITE
HOST SITE
PICNIC AREA
VISITOR CENTER

N

PACIFIC OCEAN

MAIN BEACH

To SEAL-WATCHING STATION, LAGUNA POINT

SURFWOOD SITES 108-143

WALK-IN ONLY SITES 1-10

HAUL ROAD

WEST PINEWOOD SITES 60-107

EAST PINEWOOD SITES 21-59

MILL CREEK ROAD

HS

CLEONE SITES 1-20

LAKE CLEONE

MACKERRICHER STATE PARK

To FORT BRAGG

HS

1

GETTING THERE

From Fort Bragg, go 3 miles north on CA 1 to the MacKerricher State Park entrance on the left.

GPS COORDINATES

UTM Zone (WGS84) 10S

Easting 0431967

Northing 4371330

Latitude N 39° 29' 19.9969"

Longtitude W 123° 47' 28.1184"

guided rides on the beach or in the redwoods for very reasonable prices.

The campgrounds are right by Fort Bragg, which promotes itself as the town "where prosperity reigns and where it rains prosperity." Fort Bragg (named for Braxton Bragg, a general in the Confederate Army) was first a particularly brutal Indian reservation and is now home to the Georgia-Pacific Lumber Mill. Go eat great seafood in Noyo Harbor just south of town. Try Samraat Cuisine on Main Street. A friend who served in the Peace Corps in India says he didn't have better food even in Bombay.

Go to the Mendocino Coast Botanical Gardens. The best blooms are in May, but anytime has something in season. Or ride the Skunk Train (phone [800] 866-1690) at the foot of Laurel Street. Antique railcars run 40 miles through the redwoods to Willits, crossing 30 bridges and going through two long tunnels.

11
MANCHESTER STATE PARK CAMPGROUND

HOW BEAUTIFUL! And how the wind does blow! No matter what time of year, this campground is ski-jacket country. And summer can be the worst. The winds blow so hard out of the north that you want to tie your tent to the car (seriously, bring extra rope to strategically tie your tent to nearby coyote brush and ceanothus). But when it's sunny, especially in winter or fall, Manchester State Beach can melt your heart. Nowhere is the coastline so beautiful. Nowhere does the lighthouse stand so starkly against the sea and sky. And probably nowhere are the locals as friendly as they are here.

Manchester (with a good grocery store) is a hop, skip, and a jump from the campground. Nearby Point Arena even has a community-owned first-run movie theater and playhouse. This country looks like the west coast of Wales, and the people feel like the Welsh— courteous, reserved, with a twinkle in their eye, and all balled up in wool sweaters against the weather.

The campground sites are nicely separated and set into the gorse for some privacy from the chest down. Then there's the beach. Miles and miles of sandy beach, with grassy dunes and the Pacific running off into the sky. Think ruddy. With the wind off the water, your face goes red quickly, and soon you'll look like a native.

Take the Alder Creek Trail from the campground. Round-trip is about 4 miles, and the loop should take you around two hours. The trail starts by Park Headquarters, goes past Lake Davis to the beach, and on north to Alder Creek, where there are birds and more birds (bring binoculars) around the lagoon. Look for the whistling swan. Unlike the mute swan, the whistlers hold their necks straight and bills level, and sometimes show a bright yellow spot on their black bills.

The immature swan is a light gray-brown. Since

> *Often windy and cold, Manchester State Park Campground is always breathtakingly beautiful.*

RATINGS

Beauty: ✪ ✪ ✪ ✪ ✪
Privacy: ✪ ✪ ✪ ✪
Spaciousness: ✪ ✪ ✪ ✪
Quiet: ✪ ✪ ✪ ✪ ✪
Security: ✪ ✪ ✪ ✪ ✪
Cleanliness: ✪ ✪ ✪ ✪ ✪

ADDRESS: Manchester State Park Campground P.O. Box 440 Mendocino, CA 95460

OPERATED BY: California State Parks

INFORMATION: (707) 937-5804; www.parks.ca.gov

OPEN: Year-round

SITES: 18 sites for tents or RVs, 10 environmental sites in the dunes (1-mile level walk from parking lot)

EACH SITE HAS: Picnic table, fireplace

ASSIGNMENT: First come, first served; only group site is reservable

REGISTRATION: By entrance; reserve group site by phone, (800) 444-7275, or online, www.reserve america.com

FACILITIES: Water, vault toilets, firewood for sale

PARKING: At individual site

FEE: $15; group site $90 with $7.50 nonrefundable reservation fee

ELEVATION: Sea level

RESTRICTIONS: *Pets:* On leash only
Fires: In fireplace
Alcohol: No restrictions
Vehicles: RVs up to 30 feet, trailers up to 22 feet
Other: Stay limit of 15 consecutive days, 30 days annually

the whistler is our most common swan, the chances that the swans you see in the lagoon are whistlers are pretty good. The "whistle" of the whistling swan comes from that ethereal sound the swans make when they are flying to and from the Arctic, where they nest. These swans have a seven-foot wingspan and weigh up to 20 pounds—and they need all of it for the journey. They come all that way to hang out in the "mild" Manchester Beach weather for the winter. In addition to swans, look for pelicans, godwits, killdeer, and surf scoters (a variety of sea duck).

Peaceful Alder Creek used to be famous for its "grizz"—the huge California bears that hung out around here. Imagine coming around a curve in Alder Creek and running into a mammoth grumpy grizzly bear! That would thin out the tourist herd. Fortunately for us, the last California grizz bit the dust in 1922 (so much for our state animal).

Then came the famous Alder Creek gunfight, where farmers forted up and fought off the timber company's gunfighters, who turned out to be recent graduates of San Quentin Penitentiary. After a few drunken incidents, the gunfighters wound up on a schooner bound for San Francisco, and the farmers sold out their virgin redwoods to the lumber company for peanuts. So it goes.

Pause at Alder Creek and consider the San Andreas Fault. This is where the fault comes ashore and heads down through Southern California. This area took a huge hit in the 1906 earthquake. Much of Point Arena was destroyed; fences were moved six feet—rock-and-roll time for the locals. Remember, this is why Native Americans in this region lived in temporary shelters not unlike a Kelty tent—so they could survive the big ones.

Another good hike is out to the beach and south to the mouth of the Garcia. The Manchester State Beach is a catch basin for sea debris, which accounts for the tremendous amount of driftwood found here. In fact, the beach often looks like a graveyard for driftwood. This is all good for building shelters from the howling north wind. Pass Brush Creek and pretty soon you'll come to a big lagoon and the Garcia River. Look

MAP

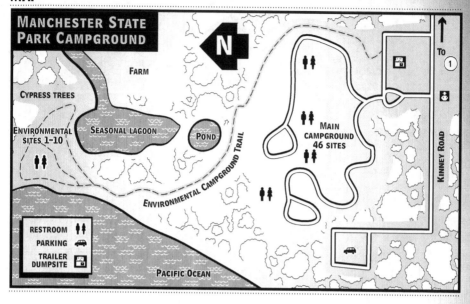

MANCHESTER STATE PARK CAMPGROUND

FARM

CYPRESS TREES

ENVIRONMENTAL SITES 1-10

SEASONAL LAGOON

POND

ENVIRONMENTAL CAMPGROUND TRAIL

MAIN CAMPGROUND 46 SITES

KINNEY ROAD

To (1)

RESTROOM
PARKING
TRAILER DUMPSITE

PACIFIC OCEAN

for many of the same bird species you saw up at Alder Creek. However, the Garcia is steelhead country. You'll want to be here at high tide in January or February—there's a prime spot called Miner Hole not far from the parking area on Miner Hole Road. Most of the anglers I've seen here wear waders and work their way downstream. Look for where the locals are fishing and follow their lead.

It's not that Manchester Beach is so cold—the swans think it's tropical—but we humanoids don't have the down feathers. We need good warm clothes because a wind-chill factor can make 50°F feel like freezing. Bring gloves—warm hands make you feel warm. Bring a sweatshirt with a hood for hanging around and sleeping in—most of your heat escapes from your head. And bring earplugs for sleeping—the flapping of the tent might keep you awake.

GETTING THERE

From Point Arena, drive 2 miles north on CA 1 past Manchester and Home Sweet Home Ranch to Kinney Road. Turn left and drive to the campground.

GPS COORDINATES

UTM Zone (WGS84) 10S
Easting 0438873
Northing 4314982
Latitude N 38° 58' 54.0983"
Longtitude W 123° 42' 20.6497"

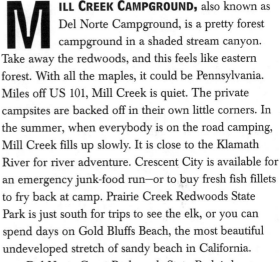

> *Feels like eastern forest camping—this is the last beautiful state park to fill up on summer weekends.*

MILL CREEK CAMPGROUND, also known as Del Norte Campground, is a pretty forest campground in a shaded stream canyon. Take away the redwoods, and this feels like eastern forest. With all the maples, it could be Pennsylvania. Miles off US 101, Mill Creek is quiet. The private campsites are backed off in their own little corners. In the summer, when everybody is on the road camping, Mill Creek fills up slowly. It is close to the Klamath River for river adventure. Crescent City is available for an emergency junk-food run—or to buy fresh fish fillets to fry back at camp. Prairie Creek Redwoods State Park is just south for trips to see the elk, or you can spend days on Gold Bluffs Beach, the most beautiful undeveloped stretch of sandy beach in California.

Del Norte Coast Redwoods State Park is huge—with 6,400 acres of redwoods, rhododendrons, wildflowers, tidepools, meadows, and beaches. This little corner of California is frontier. Lovely little Trinidad to the south is the last port of call for New Age California. Up here men can fix the truck, catch salmon, rig a crab trap, and run a chain saw. All the women call you "Honey" and sound like they mean it. Fuel for the bellies of the folks in Del Norte County (forget pronouncing the *e* on Norte) is coffee, beer, and salmon jerky.

Come prepared for wet weather. Think big tent. Big tents are better if you're cooped up for a while. You get less claustrophobic and they're easier to cook in if need be. Also consider a screen house—the mosquitoes can get pesky up here as well. Plus, on a dry night, screen houses are fun to sleep in.

Mill Creek Campground is lumberjack country. Hobbs, Wall & Company once set up a private railroad called Del Norte Southern to take the logs out of Mill Creek. The redwoods grow on such steep slopes that the timber company had to build a system of railed

RATINGS

Beauty: ✪ ✪ ✪ ✪ ✪
Privacy: ✪ ✪ ✪ ✪ ✪
Spaciousness: ✪ ✪ ✪ ✪
Quiet: ✪ ✪ ✪
Security: ✪ ✪ ✪ ✪ ✪
Cleanliness: ✪ ✪ ✪ ✪ ✪

"inclines" to the canyon and railroad below. Logs were hauled along the ridges above to an incline, where they were lowered to the canyon and railcars below.

The men did the rest of the work. They chopped the trees, limbed them, and ran the chains. It was brutal, and it gave rise to another industry—feeding 165 hungry lumberjacks down in Mill Creek three meals a day. It was serious business—each man had his seat at the table and no one could speak until the meal was over. Mammoth quantities of meat, potatoes, canned vegetables, bread, butter, and dessert were consumed. Talk about carb- and protein-loading—these boys worked 12 hours a day, ate, and slept. Look at an old photo of the jacks— not a tubby one in the bunch—thin as rails and strong as oxen. On Saturday night they left for the bars and cathouses of Crescent City, returning to Mill Creek Canyon on Monday morning to work. There were kids in the canyon, too, and a lady schoolteacher to educate them. She lived in a log cabin with a drafty roof and rode the incline down to the camp every day to teach.

Hike the Trestle Trail loop along the bed of the old Hobbs, Wall & Company logging railroad that ran beside Mill Creek. Find the trailhead just northeast of the bridge between Cascara (campsites 73 through 125) and Red Alder Campground (campsites 1 through 72). The trail heads up the hillside past big stumps and maples (the alders and maples show rich color in the fall). Cross a wooden bridge and walk along the old railbed. See how the second-growth redwoods have circled the stumps of the trees cut by the company. Half a mile down the railbed, past another bridge, look for what's left of the trestle. Stay on the trail, bearing right until you come down into Red Alder Loop by campsite 7. The whole trip is a little more than a mile.

Other trails out of Mill Creek are the Hobbs Wall Trail, the Mill Creek Trail, the Alder Basin Trail, and the Saddler Skyline Trail. Hike the Damnation Creek Trail down to the little beach with the sea stacks and tidepools. A shorter tidepool walk is the Enderts Beach Trail at the end of Enderts Beach Road. Find the road just south of Crescent City where Humboldt Road goes north. Drive out to Requa (once a Yurok village), and hike north from the end of the road.

KEY INFORMATION

ADDRESS:	Mill Creek Campground Del Norte Coast Redwoods State Park 1375 Elk Valley Road Crescent City, CA 95531
OPERATED BY:	California State Parks
INFORMATION:	(707) 464-6101, ext. 5120; www.parks.ca.gov
OPEN:	May–October
SITES:	145 sites for tents or RVs
EACH SITE HAS:	Picnic table, fireplace, food storage cabinet
ASSIGNMENT:	First come, first served; reservations recommended
REGISTRATION:	Reserve by phone, (800) 444-7275, or online, www.reserveamerica.com
FACILITIES:	Water, flush toilets, showers, wood for sale; wheelchair-accessible sites
PARKING:	At individual site
FEE:	$20; $7.50 non-refundable reservation fee
ELEVATION:	670 feet
RESTRICTIONS:	*Pets:* On leash only *Fires:* In fireplace *Alcohol:* No restrictions *Vehicles:* RVs up to 31 feet, trailers up to 27 feet *Other:* 15-day stay limit in peak season, 30-day limit in off-season; reservations recommended on summer holidays

MAP

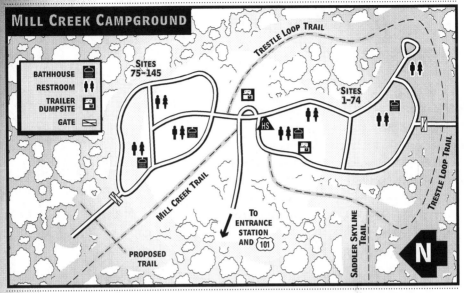

MILL CREEK CAMPGROUND

BATHHOUSE
RESTROOM
TRAILER DUMPSITE
GATE

SITES 75-145

SITES 1-74

TRESTLE LOOP TRAIL

MILL CREEK TRAIL

TRESTLE LOOP TRAIL

SADDLER SKYLINE TRAIL

To ENTRANCE STATION AND 101

PROPOSED TRAIL

N

GETTING THERE

From Crescent City, drive 9 miles south on US 101. The entrance to Mill Creek Campground is on the left. Be careful because this is on a blind curve. The campground is several miles east of US 101 on the access road—look for a sign that reads "Del Norte Campground."

Crescent City is the closest supply source. Check out the Del Norte County Historical Society Museum (phone [707] 464-3922 for hours), or the Battery Point Lighthouse. No stranger to mishap, Crescent City was hit by a tsunami, caused by the Alaskan earthquake in 1964, that killed 14 and destroyed the downtown. And a few miles offshore, the steamer *Brother Jonathan* hit a reef and 200 passengers drowned. Win some, lose some, I guess. This is a big-shouldered frontier town.

GPS COORDINATES

UTM Zone (WGS84) 10T
Easting 0406901
Northing 4613814
Latitude N 41° 40' 14.3366"
Longtitude W 124° 7' 6.1970"

13
NADELOS AND WAILAKI CAMPGROUNDS

THESE PRETTY LITTLE brother-and-sister campgrounds are right in the belly of the beast of the Lost Coast, where a fist of mountains rises straight out of the surf and black-sand beach. The terrain is so rugged that highway engineers had to route CA 1 many miles inland, leaving this huge hunk of land virtually untouched and begging to be explored. Nadelos or Wailaki campgrounds make a perfect base to do exactly that.

On top of each other, Nadelos and Wailaki are virtually the same campground. Coming off Shelter Cove Road, Nadelos is first—the eight campsites are a short walk from the parking lot and are tucked into a hill across Little Bear Creek. Half a mile south is the entrance to Wailaki, which is engineered for trailers and RVs but is wonderful for tent camping as well. Last time I was there, both campgrounds were vacant, so we stayed at Wailaki, in one of the larger campsites. Both campgrounds have water and were recently reengineered, so the sites look clean and inviting, and the pit-style toilets are immaculate.

The valley is oriented north to south, so don't expect much sunlight at either Nadelos or Wailaki, except in the middle of the day. In fact, don't expect much sunlight on the Lost Coast unless you come in September or October, the region's premium-weather months.

From October through April, the Lost Coast is one of the wettest spots on the Pacific Coast. In wet years, the Lost Coast can get up to 200 inches of rain. That's 16 feet! April and May are often windy, and the landscape is at its most lush. In June, July, and August, sunshine alternates with thick fog. Ah, but September and October are heaven. The hills are golden, and the sunsets explode across the sky.

> *A good base camp for exploring the fabulous Lost Coast. Try to come in the fall.*

RATINGS

Beauty: ✿ ✿ ✿ ✿ ✿
Privacy: ✿ ✿ ✿ ✿ ✿
Spaciousness: ✿ ✿ ✿ ✿ ✿
Quiet: ✿ ✿ ✿ ✿
Security: ✿ ✿
Cleanliness: ✿ ✿ ✿ ✿ ✿

ADDRESS: Nadelos or Wailaki
Campground
Arcata Resource Area
U.S. Bureau of Land
Management
1695 Heindon Road
Arcata, CA 95521

OPERATED BY: U.S. Department of
the Interior, Bureau
of Land Management

INFORMATION: (707) 986-5400;
www.ca.blm.gov/
arcata

OPEN: Year-round (depending on road and
weather conditions)

SITES: Nadelos has 8 tent-
only sites (entire camp
can be reserved as
group site); Wailaki
has 13 sites for tents
or RVs

EACH SITE HAS: Picnic table, fire ring

ASSIGNMENT: First come, first
served; no
reservations except
group site at Nadelos
(no reservations
Memorial Day, July 4,
Labor Day weekends)

REGISTRATION: At entrance

FACILITIES: Water, pit toilets;
wheelchair-accessible
sites at Nadelos

PARKING: At individual site

FEE: $8; $1 day-use; $85
Nadelos group site

ELEVATION: 1,840 feet

RESTRICTIONS: *Pets:* On leash only
Fires: In fire ring
Alcohol: No
restrictions
Vehicles: RVs and trailers at Wailaki only
(no hookups)
Other: 14-day stay limit;
don't leave food out;
$5 bear-canister rental

Of course, tucked into the woods at Nadelos or Wailaki, don't expect to see the sunset. You have to drive down to the beach at Shelter Cove to see that. Shelter Cove used to be a giant sheep ranch but now has been developed into a real-estate nightmare. Retirees come in, build huge houses, go crazy from the isolation of the Lost Coast, and run screaming back to civilization. So there are lots of big houses going for very few dollars at Shelter Cove.

There are wonderful beaches as well. Black Sands Beach at the north end of town basically continues 24 miles north to the mouth of the Mattole River. This is a famous hike that folks usually take from north to south because of the prevailing winds. Hikers should bring water (or a water-purifying device), a tidal schedule to time certain beaches, and camping equipment. In town, near the Pelican Landings Restaurant, find the short trail to Little Black Sands Beach, which is a favorite of the locals. And, of course, south of town past the Shelter Cove Marina and Campground is Dead Man's Beach—famous among beach people.

While you're in town, don't miss the fish and chips at the Shelter Cove Campground Deli. The fish is incredible—caught fresh every morning. The chips are thick and light. The portions are enormous. I asked for a half portion, and the tiny woman at the counter laughed. "If I can eat a whole order, so can you, big boy!" she said, and she was right. I sat outside at the picnic tables with my fish and chips and beer, with the sun setting on the whole Pacific Ocean before me.

At both Nadelos and Wailaki campgrounds, you'll spot signed trails that head west to both the Lost Coast Trail and the Hidden Valley Trail. The Hidden Valley Trail heads north 1.75 miles to the Chemise Mountain Road, where you can walk back south past the little cabins to the campgrounds. The trail south goes to Chemise Mountain (3 miles round-trip) and Whale Gulch (10 miles round-trip). Look for a herd of trans-planted Roosevelt elk along the way.

Bring water. The nearest water on the Whale Gulch Trail is at the Needle Rock visitor center 6 miles away. It's not a bad idea to stash a car or arrange a

MAP

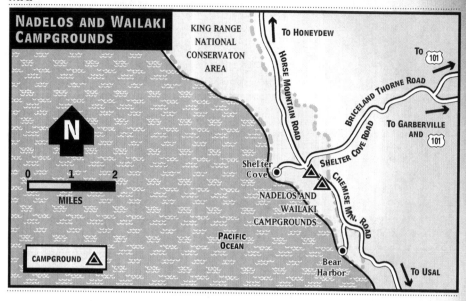

NADELOS AND WAILAKI CAMPGROUNDS

KING RANGE NATIONAL CONSERVATON AREA

To HONEYDEW

To 101

HORSE MOUNTAIN ROAD

BRICELAND THORNE ROAD

SHELTER COVE ROAD

To GARBERVILLE AND 101

Shelter Cove

NADELOS AND WAILAKI CAMPGROUNDS

CHEMISE MTN. ROAD

PACIFIC OCEAN

Bear Harbor

To USAL

N

0   1   2
MILES

CAMPGROUND △

---

pick-up at the visitor center for the trip back. (To reach Needle Rock from the campgrounds, head south on Chemise Mountain Road to Four Corners, then go right on Briceland Road to Needle Rock.)

For a grueling but fun road-trip, turn south on Usal Road at Four Corners and drive down to Usal Beach and CA 1. Phone the Sinkyone Wilderness State Park at (707) 986-7711 to get a reading on the road conditions. Impassable in winter, this road hasn't changed much since Jack London and his wife, Charmian, came up in a wagon in 1911.

GETTING THERE

From Redway (by Garberville) on US 101, drive 22 miles west on Shelter Cove Road. Go 2 miles south on Chemise Mountain Road to Nadelos Campground, then another 0.5 miles south to Wailaki Campground.

GPS COORDINATES

Wailaki
UTM Zone (WGS84) 10T
Easting 0414421
Northing 4430260
Latitude N 40° 1' 5.5562"
Longtitude W 124° 0' 10.1774"

GPS COORDINATES

Nadelos
UTM Zone (WGS84) 10T
Easting 0414140
Northing 4430572
Latitude N 40° 1' 15.5713"
Longtitude W 124° 0' 22.1761"

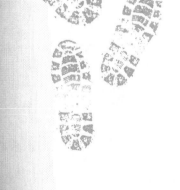

> *Patrick's Point Campground has everything—beauty, sea lions, a Native American village, and hot clam chowder nearby.*

MOST BEAUTIFUL OF ALL California's state parks, Patrick's Point is full of enchanted Sitka-spruce groves and dizzying cliffs running down to ancient sea stacks, sea lions, and the foaming green Pacific. The three campground loops in the park, Agate, Penn, and Abalone, are under trees— the campsites nestled in bracken fern, sword fern, and salmonberry. The Sitkas, with their silver moss, crinkled bark, and golden cones, loom out of the mist. Each site is private, secluded, and special. On the beach, find agates and sometimes jade. Surf fish for perch and flounder. With the Yurok village of Sumeg in the park, and Trinidad nearby with the marine lab and party fishing boats, there's lots to do with kids.

Take the Rim Trail to get a sense of the headlands. Accessible from various places, the trail goes 2 miles around the promontory, passing little trails to Palmers Point, Abalone Point, Rocky Point, Patrick's Point, Wedding Rock, and Mussel Rocks. By the time you take all these spur trails, the trip is more like 4 miles. Wedding Rock is a good place to look for whales during the season.

Head to Palmer's Point and climb down to the tidepool area. Look for sea lions and harbor seals. The sea lions are bigger than the seals, without spots, and their buff-to-brown hide looks black when it is wet. Sea lions are the fastest swimmers—up to 25 mph when pressed. They can descend to 450 feet and stay submerged for 20 minutes. They use sonar to get around and find their prey.

Hike down to Agate Beach where the agate finding is easiest after a high tide. The best hunting, though, is after a winter storm. The agates found here are unpolished and look just like little white-and-bluish quartz stones. Take them home and put them in a bottle with oil so they always look wet and pretty. Keep hiking for

RATINGS

Beauty: ✿ ✿ ✿ ✿ ✿
Privacy: ✿ ✿ ✿ ✿ ✿
Spaciousness: ✿ ✿ ✿ ✿
Quiet: ✿ ✿ ✿
Security: ✿ ✿ ✿ ✿ ✿
Cleanliness: ✿ ✿ ✿ ✿ ✿

2 miles and come to Humboldt Lagoons State Park. These lagoons are the sand-drowned mouths of streams. Spits of wave-borne sand form across their outlets to dam up the streams until the ocean cuts a floodgate through. Check out the dunes for beach pea, salt grass, verbena, and sea rocket. On the shore is more Sitka spruce, red alder, and redwood. This was prime Yurok Native American country.

The Yuroks moved between fishing and hunting camps. They trapped elk in deep pits covered with branches and dirt, and they speared sea lions by painting their own bodies dark and wriggling up close enough for the kill. They netted ducks and geese and gill-netted salmon. The women gathered acorns and leached them, and made bread. Dried eel was a specialty (a big hit with hungry European explorers). Abalone was an everyday staple, as well as edible seaweed. The Yuroks lived well.

At the foot of the lagoons is Big Lagoon County Park, with a boat ramp for canoers, kayakers, and windsurfers. Consider the tent camping here for another trip or if Patrick's Point is jammed up. You are at water ground zero just off the Big Lagoon. The tent pitches are grassy sand. There's good camping (no reservations), but not much of the cover privacy that Patrick's Point has in spades. I talked to the ranger there who said the fishing is pretty slim until the ocean cuts through the dunes. Then you get steelhead, sea-run cutthroat trout, sharks, flounders, and so on. To drive to Big Lagoon County Park from Patrick's Point, just go 1 mile north on US 101. Turn left at Big Lagoon Road and follow the signs.

Another good trip is to nearby Trinidad. Everyone likes the Humboldt State Lab and Aquarium (open weekdays 9 a.m. to 5 p.m.). Sir Francis Drake once anchored at this old whaling town, which now offers peerless clam chowder and crab sandwiches at the Seascape Restaurant down on the Trinidad Wharf. The fish and crab come off the fishing boats and directly through the kitchen door of Seascape.

Come here in July and go for salmon. There are charter and party boats available, and the fish are sometimes close enough for small boats. A word of

KEY INFORMATION

ADDRESS:	Patrick's Point State Park Campground 4150 Patrick's Point Drive Trinidad, CA 95570
OPERATED BY:	California State Parks
INFORMATION:	(707) 677-3570; www.parks.ca.gov
OPEN:	Year-round
SITES:	124 sites for tents or RVs, 2 group sites, enviromental camp for hikers and cyclists
EACH SITE HAS:	Picnic table, fireplace, food-storage cabinet
ASSIGNMENT:	Assigned by ranger
REGISTRATION:	By entrance; reserve by phone, (800) 444-7275, or online, www.reserve america.com
FACILITIES:	Water, flush toilets, coin-operated showers, firewood for sale
PARKING:	At individual site
FEE:	$20; $6 extra vehicle; $7.50 nonrefundable reservation fee
ELEVATION:	100 feet
RESTRICTIONS:	*Pets:* On leash only in campground, not on trails *Fires:* In fireplace *Alcohol:* No restrictions *Vehicles:* RVs up to 31 feet *Other:* Reservations recommended on holidays and summer weekends; stay limit: 15 days in summer. 30 days annually; new group area completed in 2004

MAP

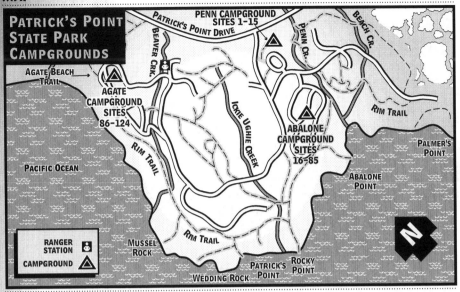

PATRICK'S POINT STATE PARK CAMPGROUNDS

PENN CAMPGROUND SITES 1-15

PATRICK'S POINT DRIVE

BEAVER CRK.

PENN CRK.

BEACH CR.

AGATE BEACH TRAIL

AGATE CAMPGROUND SITES 86-124

IXIE UGHIE CREEK

RIM TRAIL

RIM TRAIL

ABALONE CAMPGROUND SITES 16-85

PALMER'S POINT

PACIFIC OCEAN

ABALONE POINT

RANGER STATION

CAMPGROUND

MUSSEL ROCK

RIM TRAIL

WEDDING ROCK

PATRICK'S POINT

ROCKY POINT

GETTING THERE

From Trinidad, go 5 miles north on US 101 to the Patrick's Point State Park entrance on the left.

GPS COORDINATES

UTM Zone (WGS84) 10T
Easting 0402636
Northing 4554516
Latitude N 41° 8' 10.0211"
Longtitude W 124° 9' 36.2698"

warning though: this coast is notorious for fogging in, so watch your navigation or you'll end up in Hawaii.

No luck fishing? Stop at Katy's Smokehouse on Edwards Street across from the Trinidad Memorial Lighthouse to buy fish or crab to take back to camp. When the Dungeness come in November, Katy's is crab-lovers' heaven, and her smoked albacore is incomparable.

The Yuroks revered Patrick's Point and believed that the spirit of the porpoises lived here and that the seven sea stacks were the last earthly abode of the immortals. Patrick Beegan, an Irishman who came here in 1851, just liked the wild Indian potatoes (lily bulbs) that grew here, hence the name Patrick's Point.

THERE'S NO SHORTAGE of incredible campsites along the Northern California coast, but Pomo Canyon, a walk-in campground nestled in a small redwood canyon just over a low ridge from the ocean, is unique. Since only tents are permitted and camping gear must be hauled in from the parking lot, Pomo Canyon is perfect for minimalists or backpackers ironing out the kinks for future treks. All the sites are completely shaded by the redwood forest. A few sites are scattered near a creek along the canyon floor, where redwood sorrel, stream violet, and trillium bloom in spring. The other campsites, which perch on a hillside above the canyon, have a limited amount of level space for tents, although some visitors have carved tent shelves into the hillsides (park staff doesn't condone this). It's a little more than a 0.1-mile level walk to the most remote sites: 17 through 21. Sites 1 through 6 are accessed via Dr. David Joseph Memorial Trail (informally know as Pomo Canyon Trail), which climbs uphill out of the campground to coastal scrub on the flanks of Red Hill, then drifts easily downhill to Shell Beach. This 5.5-mile round-trip hike can be combined with hours of beach strolling along the Sonoma Coast State Beach coastline, which stretches 17 miles, from Bodega Head to a view point 4 miles north of Jenner.

Pomo Canyon is one of four top-notch campgrounds nearby, all part of the Sonoma Coast State Beach system. The second environmental campground, Willow Creek, is just down the road (you'll pass the entrance on the way to Pomo Canyon) and fronts the Russian River. Willow Creek has 11 walk-in sites, with a mixture of sunshine and shade. The campground does not have water, and traffic noise from CA 116 filters over to the campground, but you might consider Willow Creek if you want a break from Pomo Canyon's cool, dark redwood canyon.

> *Pomo Canyon offers no-frills camping in a cool, shaded redwood canyon.*

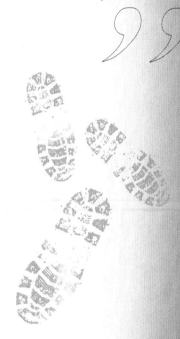

RATINGS

Beauty: ✰ ✰ ✰ ✰ ✰
Privacy: ✰ ✰ ✰
Spaciousness: ✰ ✰ ✰
Quiet: ✰ ✰ ✰ ✰
Security: ✰ ✰
Cleanliness: ✰ ✰ ✰ ✰

KEY INFORMATION

ADDRESS: Pomo Canyon
Campground
Sonoma County
State Beach
3095 CA 1
Bodega Bay, CA
94923

OPERATED BY: California State
Parks

INFORMATION: (707) 875-3483;
www.parks.ca.gov

OPEN: April 1–
November 30

SITES: 20 tent-only sites

EACH SITE HAS: Fire ring, picnic
table

ASSIGNMENT: First come, first
served; no
reservations

REGISTRATION: At the self-
registration station
at the campground
entrance

FACILITIES: Drinking water,
vault toilets

PARKING: At lot; walk in to
sites

FEE: $10 night

ELEVATION: 140 feet

RESTRICTIONS: *Pets:* Dogs are not
allowed on trails or
in campground
Fires: In established
pits/rings only
Alcohol: No
restrictions
Vehicles: Camping in
vehicle in parking
lot not permitted
Other: 8 people maxi-
mum per campsite.
Stay on trails to pro-
tect the fragile red-
wood forest.

The other two campgrounds, Wrights Beach and Bodega Dunes, are open to trailers and RVs and are very popular summer destinations, with all the amenities of modern camping, including flush toilets and (at Bodega Dunes) showers. At Wrights Beach, sites 0 through 9 are right on the beach, and the other 20 spots are a short walk. At Bodega Dunes, the campground's namesake mounds of sand sprawl between the beach and the campground.

The Sonoma Coast is particularly popular in summer, when tourists roam the length of winding CA 1 soaking up the sunshine and ocean views. Fog occasionally hangs about near the coast in July and August, when the last wildflowers of the year, includ-ing buckwheat, lizardtail, and yarrow, draw many colorful dragonflies and butterflies—look for mylitta crescent, California buckeye, and small blues flutter-ing about. Folks who love exploring the outdoors in the Bay Area rave about September and October camping, when the weather is warm and clear, and kids are back in school, so campsites are less crowded.

Nearby Guerneville, an outpost on the Russian River, is a small, low-key resort town that provides refuge from city heat and features a jazz festival in summer. With a big Safeway supermarket and small shops where you can buy coffee, Guerneville is the logical stop for ice-chest supplies. There are some small wineries in western Sonoma County, but the area immediately surrounding Pomo Canyon is pri-marily coastal cattle ranches, forest, and parkland. Bodega Bay, Jenner, and Occidental are within driv-ing distance and have a handful of restaurants (but no major supermarkets), and the tiny hamlet of Free-stone is host to Wildflour, a fantastic bakery (open Friday through Monday) with exceptional breads, scones, and focaccia. If you do go out exploring by car, note that past the campground Willow Creek Road eventually becomes a dirt logging road—Coleman Valley Road is narrow but paved.

MAP

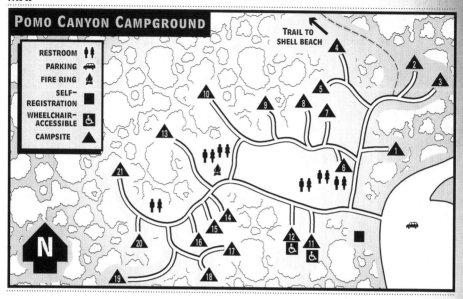

POMO CANYON CAMPGROUND

TRAIL TO
SHELL BEACH

RESTROOM
PARKING
FIRE RING
SELF–
REGISTRATION
WHEELCHAIR–
ACCESSIBLE
CAMPSITE

N

GETTING THERE

From US 101 north of Santa
Rosa in Sonoma County, exit
on River Road. Drive west
on River Road 27 miles, to
the junction with CA 1. Turn
left and drive south
0.3 miles, then turn left onto
Willow Creek Road. Drive
2.5 miles to the signed campground road, then turn right
and continue a final
0.5 miles to the parking lot at
the end of the road.

GPS COORDINATES

UTM Zone (WGS84) 10S

Easting 0492462

Northing 4254200

Latitude N 38° 26' 9.7476"

Longtitude W 123° 5' 10.9354"

> *Sits beside an azure gem of a cove next to the "jewel of the north coast," the town of Mendocino.*

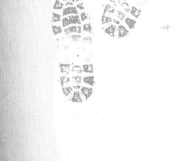

THANK **G**OD FOR **F.D.R.** and the New Deal, or we wouldn't have Russian Gulch State Park and the soaring arched concrete bridge that spans the gulch. What a pretty little campground! Take a left just after the bridge, and circle down a curved one-lane access road to the campground in the canyon and the beach across the stream under the bridge. The beach is all white sandbars, narrow blue water, soaring black cliffs spotted white, and green headlands. There is safe swimming here, and an easy launch for kayaks or inflatables.

The campground threads its way up the ferned canyon, with sites on either side of the access road. Cozy, mossy, and primal—that's what you feel tucked into a tent under the giant ferns, alders, redwoods, and hemlocks. Come here to sun on a safe beach. Fish for rockfish. Hike the Fern Canyon Trail. Hike the South Trail to Mendocino, where you can eat world-class food; shop till you drop; and hang with the rich, famous, and everyone in between.

Who named Russian Gulch? Nobody remembers, but local folks think the Russian fur hunters used to store bales of furs here in the otter- and seal-slaughtering days of the early 1800s. The Russians operated out of Fort Ross down the coast, and used Eskimo hunters in *baidarkas* (sealskin kayaks) to do the stalking and killing. The local Pomo Indians, who knew something about the sea and the seals themselves (stalking them by painting themselves dark and pretending to be seals to get close enough for a kill), were amazed by the Eskimos' skill in using their kayaks for the hunt. However, after the seals were mostly dead, the Russians packed up and headed home, leaving the Mendocino coast and the surviving Pomos easy pickings for a motley crew of forty-niners who followed the wreck of the *Frolic*.

RATINGS

Beauty: ✪ ✪ ✪ ✪ ✪
Privacy: ✪
Spaciousness: ✪ ✪
Quiet: ✪ ✪
Security: ✪ ✪ ✪ ✪
Cleanliness: ✪ ✪ ✪ ✪

The two-masted clipper ship named *Frolic* sank off of Russian Gulch in 1850 with a hull full of Chinese silks and gewgaws. Henry Meigs sent his boys from San Francisco to salvage the wreck, but they found only happy Pomo Native American women wearing skirts of Chinese silk and jewelry fashioned from oriental beads. Inevitably, Meigs heard about the huge redwoods in these parts and immediately sent a steam sawmill up to Mendocino to start ripping boards to build San Francisco, shore up gold mines in the Sierra Nevada, and make railroad ties for the Transcontinental Railway. The place boomed, with dozens of bars and hotels to entertain the hard-partying lumberjacks.

After that, Mendocino boomed and busted and finally emerged around 1960 as the "jewel of the north coast"—a pretty little town full of arts, culture, great grub, scenic splendor, and a potpourri of Victorian gothics, New England saltboxes, and false-front Western houses. I love Mendocino. People rag on it for being too cutsie, but I love it just the way it is—perfect for a couple of days of hanging out. The campground is an easy walk from town—just head up the South Trail where it leaves the beach road opposite the group camp. You come up over the bluffs, then walk along CA 1 before taking the first right toward Mendocino.

Back at camp, hike the Fern Canyon Trail. This is a 6-mile round-trip trail that allows cyclists as far as the start of the Waterfall Loop. Head east through the campground. Look for nettles, salmonberry, and nightshade down by the creek, and alder, hazel, and laurel by the trail. After half a mile, you'll begin to see redwoods. At 1.5 miles there are some picnic tables. Beyond here, no bicycles are allowed. Hike up to the falls and admire their splendor. Then take the loop around to the right, back to the picnic tables, and retrace the trail back to the campground.

Another good walk is the Headland Trail. This 1-mile trail circles the park's north headland, showing off the incredible surf-carved rocks and cliffs. At the southwest end, look for a blowhole fed by a sea cave. Big waves blast up through the blowhole. Inland, look for the punch bowl where the roof of another cave collapsed. Plants hang over the rim, but the sea

MAP

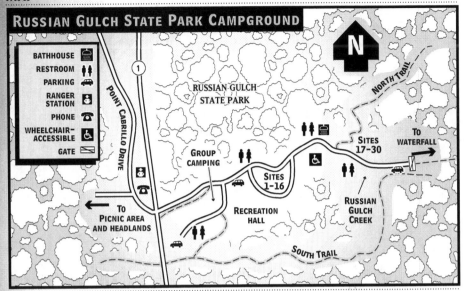

RUSSIAN GULCH STATE PARK CAMPGROUND

BATHHOUSE
RESTROOM
PARKING
RANGER STATION
PHONE
WHEELCHAIR-ACCESSIBLE
GATE

RUSSIAN GULCH STATE PARK

POINT CABRILLO DRIVE

NORTH TRAIL

SITES 17-30

TO WATERFALL

GROUP CAMPING

SITES 1-16

RUSSIAN GULCH CREEK

TO PICNIC AREA AND HEADLANDS

RECREATION HALL

SOUTH TRAIL

GETTING THERE

From Mendocino, go 2 miles north on CA 1 to the campground entrance on the left.

GPS COORDINATES

UTM Zone (WGS84) 10S
Easting 0431579
Northing 4350491
Latitude N 39° 18' 3.9601"
Longtitude W 123° 47' 36.6899"

comes in through a small opening and washes the floor clean.

Good fun is canoeing the Big River. Phone Catch-a-Canoe & Bicycles, Too!, at (707) 937-0273, to rent watercraft which allow you to see seals, ducks, ospreys, and other wild critters. The Big River is an estuary, which means it's tidal, so you'll want to go upriver when the tide is coming in and downriver when the tide is going out. Go back to the jolly folks at Catch-a-Canoe and rent bicycles for a run up Little Lake Road to Caspar Orchard Road and back.

While camping at Russian Gulch, shop at Mendosa's and buy cheese at the deli that's kitty-cornered from Mendosa's. Don't forget to grab a burger at Meno Burgers, nearby on Lansing Street (the veggie burger is heartily recommended).

17
TISH TANG
CAMPGROUND

TISH TANG IS A CAMPGROUND in the Hoopa Valley Indian Reservation, surrounded by Six Rivers National Forest. The mighty Trinity River calls out the siren song here, luring campers to a rocky-banked cool river and lulling them to sleep at night with the soothing murmur of white noise provided by the river.

To reach the campground, turn off CA 96 and descend a steep, sharply switchbacking paved road. As you enter the campground and bear left onto the one-way road, the first series of sites on the left back up onto the forested hillside. All sites in the campground are at least partially shaded, but these offer the most tree cover. The group campsite is on the right about halfway through the campground and offers a large, grassy open area for multiple tents. Sites on the back stretch of the road offer the easiest access to the river, but from any of the sites at Tish Tang, the Trinity is mere moments away.

There are two access paths to the river: one a trail departing between sites 25 and 27, and the other a gravel road that descends to the beach from a small parking area just outside the campground. In the heart of summer, the campground and day-use area are popular with folks looking for some cool river relief from soaring temperatures. Fishing for steelhead and salmon is popular, and a rafting outfit in Willow Creek offers numerous whitewater day-trip expeditions and multi-day campout trips in the area, along the Trinity and Klamath rivers (contact Bigfoot Rafting Company, P.O. Box 729, Willow Creek, CA 95573; phone (530) 629-2263 or (800) 722-2223; **www.caladventures .com/BigFootRafting.htm**).

It's a majestic sight, the Trinity—a wide, fast-moving river flowing north toward the Klamath River. The campground's namesake, Tish Tang Creek, spills

> *It's all about the Trinity River at Tish Tang, where from your campsite it's a brief walk to a gravel beach.*

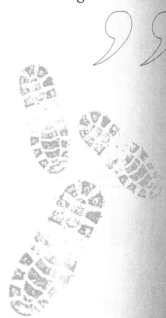

RATINGS

Beauty: ☆ ☆ ☆
Privacy: ☆ ☆ ☆ ☆
Spaciousness: ☆ ☆ ☆ ☆
Quiet: ☆ ☆ ☆ ☆
Security: ☆ ☆ ☆
Cleanliness: ☆ ☆ ☆ ☆

ADDRESS:	Tish Tang Campground Hoopa Valley Tribal Council Forestry Department P.O. Box 1368 Hoopa, CA 95546
OPERATED BY:	Hoopa Valley Tribal Council
INFORMATION:	Hoopa Valley Tribal Council, Forestry Department, (530) 625-4284
OPEN:	Late May– mid-October
SITES:	40 sites for tents and RVs up to 50 feet
EACH SITES HAS:	Picnic table, fire pit
ASSIGNMENT:	First come, first served; reservations recommended
REGISTRATION:	At camp host station if staffed; if not, camp host will come around to collect fee; reserve sites by phone at (530) 625-4284
FACILITIES:	Drinking water, vault toilets, river access
PARKING:	At individual site
FEE:	$10
ELEVATION:	300 feet
RESTRICTIONS:	*Pets:* Dogs on leash *Fires:* In established pits or rings only *Alcohol:* No restrictions *Vehicles:* $5 second-vehicle fee *Other:* Reservations made up to 3 weeks in advance

into the Trinity from the east, on the north side of the beach. When we camped here in June, the water was still quite cold and signs warned of the dangerously swift currents—swimming is not advised until July, when the water slows down and warms up. The beach area is very rocky, so if you want to lounge about, the most comfortable option is a chair rather than a blanket. There aren't a lot of terrestrial activities in the immediate area; again, it's all about the river.

In this natural setting, you don't have to work to experience nature—it's all around, and all you need do is become aware if it. Small lizards rule the campground, and you'll hear them scuttling about in the bushes. Birds are common, both in the campground and around the river, where we watched an osprey silently drop to the water and catch a fish, all in one graceful motion. California sister and swallowtail butterflies floated in the afternoon sunshine. Lucky campers may see bald eagles, otters, and beavers.

Willow Creek is a convenient last stop for campers headed to Tish Tang, offering basic camping amenities including gas, groceries, and a few restaurants.

As you drive to Tish Tang from the coast, you seem to be heading deep into the mountains, but most of the climbing and descending cancels each other out, and in the end you gain only about 300 feet in elevation. It gets good and hot at Tish Tang, so if you want cooler summer temperatures, you'll have to drive farther into the higher forests of Shasta-Trinity National Forest.

The campground was in a bit of disarray when we visited, shortly after the season's opening date. New vault toilets were being installed, and we felt a bit like guests who arrived at a party before the hosts are ready. The place feels somewhat raw; even though camp hosts are on the premises some of the time, there was a relaxed atmosphere that may not appeal to all campers. There were a few little maintenance issues (some of the fire pits were missing grills, and others were broken). Big, old oaks, madrone, pine, and Douglas fir, and a thick understory of shrubs (including plenty of poison oak) are largely ungroomed, resulting in what we call a tish tangle. We've heard that the

MAP

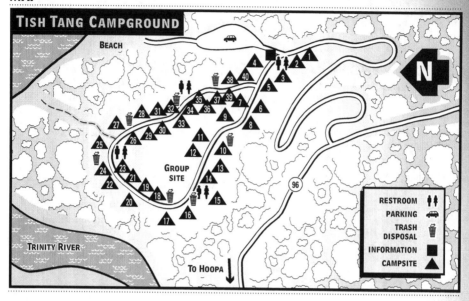

beach gets some visitation from folks who prefer to sunbath and swim in the buff. All in all, Tish Tang is a fine destination for anyone, but we think it may appeal most to campers who like their camping a little rough around the edges.

GETTING THERE

From Arcata on US 101 in Humboldt County, turn east onto CA 299. Drive east 40 miles to the town of Willow Creek, then turn left onto CA 96, signed to Hoopa. Drive north 8 miles, then turn right at the Tish Tang Campground sign. Continue downhill a short distance on the twisty road, to a fork in the road. Proceed to the left, into the campground.

GPS COORDINATES

UTM Zone (WGS84) 10T

Easting 0446353

Northing 4541498

Latitude N 41° 1' 22.5301"

Longtitude W 123° 38' 17.1708"

18
TREE OF HEAVEN
CAMPGROUND

> *Tree of Heaven Campground is good for lawn sports, river rafting, fishing, and touring at nearby Yreka.*

THE **TREE OF HEAVEN CAMPGROUND** comes as a stunning surprise. One moment you are driving along the Klamath in high sage country. You pass an old-time girder bridge (Ash Creek Bridge), sweep around a curve, and see the Forest Service sign to the Tree of Heaven Campground. The entry drive drops suddenly down to the river, and there you are at the Tree of Heaven Campground, and you suddenly feel like you've been invited to an English garden party. All over there's green, tended grass. The campsites are on grass. There's room for baseball, and in the day-use area you'll find horseshoes, an open-pit barbecue, and a volleyball court with a net in tournament shape. Everything is neat and pruned. The wood-for-sale pile by the host trailer is squared away. The campers look well groomed. Even the campers' lap dogs are well maintained and strut around Tree of Heaven on their leads like little British marines.

The Klamath rolls by the campground like a watery muscle. Most campers swim right in front of the camp off the boat launch. Here the river runs pretty slowly, but everybody keeps a close eye on any kids, pets, or poor swimmers, because this water is headed for the Pacific Ocean. Fishing can be great. One ranger I talked to said he was catching fish right and left at Tree of Heaven in late September. Last time I was through there, I was told the fish were running but nobody was catching anything yet. A lady ranger said the salmon were pretty beat up by the time they get that far, but her kids always catch good-tasting steelhead trout.

There are hikes around Tree of Heaven, including an interpretive hike near the day-use area. Take the Tree of Heaven Trail that heads down by the river about 2 miles. It takes you to a good fishing place. But

RATINGS

Beauty: ☆ ☆ ☆ ☆ ☆
Privacy: ☆ ☆ ☆ ☆
Spaciousness: ☆ ☆ ☆ ☆ ☆
Quiet: ☆ ☆ ☆ ☆ ☆
Security: ☆ ☆ ☆ ☆ ☆
Cleanliness: ☆ ☆ ☆ ☆ ☆

to really step out, you need to get in your car and head back toward I-5. Turn right on Ash Creek Bridge, which you passed on the way in. A mostly dirt road runs west down the south side of the Klamath. This is good hiking (as long as your dogs last) and great mountain biking. The road winds around with the river until it hits Walker Bridge about 25 miles downstream. On the way, you'll pass Humbug Creek Road, which is worth a look—assuming you're on your mountain bike and don't mind a climb, of course. By Walker Bridge on CA 96 is the Oak Knoll Ranger Station, so you can use the phone, beg for help, try to hitch a ride, or steel yourself for the climb back up to Tree of Heaven Campground.

The name of the game here is rafting. It's best to phone the Ranger Station a week or so in advance to get the name of a reputable rafting outfitter and arrange a trip. Locals, of course, know the waters and use their own rafts. I firmly believe that discretion for strangers in these parts is the better part of valor. Spending a little money upfront can save you a lot of grief later—especially if you bring your family along. The outfitters have helmets and life vests. Get it right the first time, and then maybe come back the next year with your own stuff.

Yreka (pronounce the *Y* then say "reka," or be roundly mocked by the locals) is a major draw only 15 minutes away. The trick is not to get on I-5 when going to and from Yreka. Not only is the exit confusing, but you lose all the sense of "being" in Yreka or in Tree of Heaven. Yreka is a wonderful little town that was founded back in 1851 by Abraham Thompson, who watched in amazement as his grazing mules brought up flecks of gold tangled in the roots of the grass. In six weeks, 2,000 miners arrived, and soon there were 27 saloons in town (first things first!). Now there's a good sports bar on the corner of Miner and Main streets.

In the Siskiyou County Museum, Yreka has the best small-museum exhibit of Native American life and crafts I've ever seen. Then there are the eye-popping nuggets in the courthouse, all the incredible Victorian houses (walk, don't drive), the Blue Goose train that steams through the Shasta Valley to Montague and

KEY INFORMATION

ADDRESS:	Tree of Heaven Campground Klamath National Forest Scott River Ranger District 11263 North CA 3 Fort Jones, CA 96032-9702
OPERATED BY:	U.S. Forest Service
INFORMATION:	(530) 468-5351; www.fs.fed.us/r5/klamath
OPEN:	Year-round; hosted May–October
SITES:	20; 1 wheelchair-accessible site
EACH SITE HAS:	Picnic table, fireplace
ASSIGNMENT:	First come, first served; reservations must be made up to 3 weeks in advance
REGISTRATION:	By entrance; reserve by phone at (530) 468-5331
FACILITIES:	Water, vault toilets
PARKING:	At individual site
FEE:	$10
ELEVATION:	2,100 feet
RESTRICTIONS:	*Pets:* On leash only *Fires:* In fireplace *Alcohol:* No restrictions *Vehicles:* Small RVs only *Other:* Check weather conditions and water availability; no Off-Highway Vehicle use, no livestock allowed; 14-day stay limit

MAP

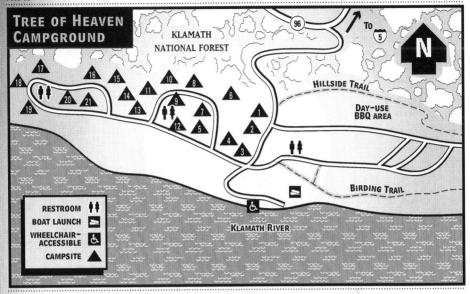

TREE OF HEAVEN CAMPGROUND

KLAMATH NATIONAL FOREST

96

To 5

N

HILLSIDE TRAIL

DAY-USE BBQ AREA

BIRDING TRAIL

KLAMATH RIVER

RESTROOM	👫
BOAT LAUNCH	🛥
WHEELCHAIR-ACCESSIBLE	♿
CAMPSITE	▲

GETTING THERE

Drive about 10 miles north of Yreka on CA 263. Turn left (west) on CA 96. Pass the Ash Creek Bridge. Look for the Tree of Heaven Campground sign a few miles farther on the left. Be careful on the turn. Or drive 10 miles north on I-5 to CA 96. Exit and go west on CA 96 to the campground on the left, after passing the Ash Creek Bridge.

GPS COORDINATES

UTM Zone (WGS84) 10T
Easting 0528275
Northing 4631189
Latitude N 41° 49' 55.5022"
Longtitude W 122° 39' 34.1318"

back again (phone [530] 842-4146 for a schedule of the different runs), and all of the very friendly people.

Tired of camping? Spend an inexpensive but very comfortable night in the Wayside Inn. Right next door is a diner that serves up a whopping good breakfast for just a pinch of gold dust.

The tree that gives the campground its name is a Chinese tree (*Ailanthus altissima*), commonly called the Tree of Heaven. Chinese laborers planted the tree by gold mines and along railroad tracks. Known as a weed tree because it spreads by root suckers and "airplane propeller" seeds, the Tree of Heaven is attractive and indestructible.

19
VAN DAMME STATE PARK CAMPGROUNDS

VAN **DAMME STATE PARK** lies along the most beautiful stretch of coast in America, where it doesn't snow during the wintertime (unlike Maine). There is a sandy beach where folks actually dare swim, whales, abalone, antique shops, a pygmy forest, fabulous restaurants, and tent pitches on moss so soft you'll sleep like a baby. This is a well-run, friendly park. There are rangers, docents, and a campground host. Open all year, Van Damme is a park for all seasons.

Charles Van Damme was a Flemish kid who busted a gut working in a sawmill in Little River after the Civil War. He went on to operate the Richmond–San Rafael ferry, but he left his heart in Little River. When he finally got some bucks together, he bought 40 acres there and later willed them to the State of California. That land became the core of Van Damme State Park— now 2,163 acres of beach and upland.

Well before Charles, Native Americans lived along here as far back as 10,000 years. Of course, in those days, the sea level was 250 feet lower than it is today, so the shore where they gathered food was about 2 miles west in the briny deep, and the grassy headlands where we hike today were then pine forest.

Around 1587, a Spaniard on a galleon named this coast Mendocino for his friend back home—Antonio de Mendosa. A couple hundred years later the Russians came for the sea-otter pelts and were soon followed by the padres and the forty-niners, who were smitten by the beauty of the place and settled here after driving out the defenseless Pomo Native Americans. When Smeaton Chase, the eccentric English traveler, came through in 1911, he described the area as "such headlands, black and wooded, such purple seas, such vivid blaze of spray, such fiords and islets . . ." and the town of Little River itself as "a pretty, straggling village of

> *Come for the ocean, the whales, the pygmy forest, and nearby Mendocino.*

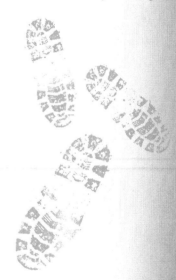

RATINGS

Beauty: ✪ ✪ ✪ ✪ ✪
Privacy: ✪
Spaciousness: ✪ ✪ ✪ ✪
Quiet: ✪
Security: ✪ ✪ ✪
Cleanliness: ✪ ✪ ✪ ✪ ✪

ADDRESS: Van Damme State Park P.O. Box 440 Mendocino, CA 94560

OPERATED BY: California State Parks

INFORMATION: (707) 937-5804; www.parks.ca.gov

OPEN: Year-round

SITES: 74 sites for tents or RVs, 10 hike-in sites in Fern Canyon; also a group site for up to 50 people

EACH SITE HAS: Picnic table, fireplace

ASSIGNMENT: First come, first served; reservations recommended

REGISTRATION: By ranger; reserve by phone, (800) 444-7275, or online, www.reserve america.com

FACILITIES: Wi-Fi access near visitor center, water, flush toilets, hot showers, wood for sale

PARKING: At individual site

FEE: $25 ($20 off-season); $7.50 nonrefundable reservation fee

ELEVATION: 15 feet

RESTRICTIONS: *Pets:* On leash only in campground, not allowed on trails *Fires:* In fireplace *Alcohol:* No restrictions *Vehicles:* RVs up to 35 feet *Other:* Reservations required April–October; 2-week stay limit; up to 8 people per site

high gabled houses with quaint dormers and windows, and red roses clambering all about."

Little River is still pretty, and fun. Find the Little River Golf & Tennis Club—open to the public—and food and spirits at the Little River Restaurant and the Little River Inn. Or go a mile or so north to the much-fabled Mendocino, home to many restaurants, shops, and colorful locals. You may recognize it as Cabot Cove, Maine, the hometown of the fictional character Jessica Fletcher of *Murder, She Wrote.*

Watch for whales. It's best to look between December and May, in the morning, when the sea is calm. The gray whales migrate from the Bering Sea to Baja California, where they give birth to their 1,500-pound calves. Mama weighs in at about 30 tons. Look for them blowing water before diving down 100 feet for three or four minutes. To get a closer look at these behemoths, take a whale-watching boat out of Noyo Harbor in Fort Bragg (10 miles to the north).

There are a couple of decent hikes in the park. Head up the Fern Canyon Trail, which starts as a fire road at the east end of Lower Campground. Pass sword fern and redwood, hemlock, and fir along the canyon. By Little River grow alder, salmonberry, and thimbleberry. After 2 miles, the fire road ends (bicycles are allowed this far), and the trail goes deeper into Fern Canyon through Douglas fir, redwood, and a plethora of fern. The trail heads out of the canyon and circles back to the right, passing a redwood stump about ten feet in diameter.

When you reach a junction with a dirt road, you can go left to the pygmy forest, where old-growth trees have one-inch diameters and heights of four feet! Why? The soil is hard and mineralized, so the cypress and Bolander pine are stunted but produce an impressive crop of pinecones. In between these trees, look for tan oak and rhododendron, as well as blackberries and wax myrtle. Just beyond the pygmy forest is the Little River Airport Road, which heads back to Little River and CA 1. You can catch a ride back to camp, or head back through the pygmy forest to the trail you hiked in on.

Back at campground central, take a stroll around the Bog Trail loop. This half-mile walk begins near the

MAP

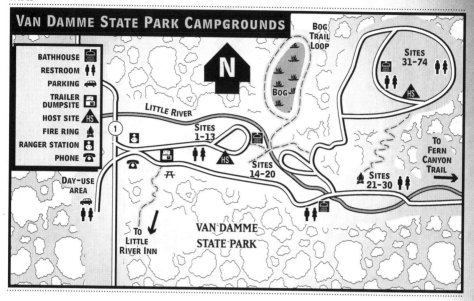

VAN DAMME STATE PARK CAMPGROUNDS

BATHHOUSE
RESTROOM
PARKING
TRAILER DUMPSITE
HOST SITE
FIRE RING
RANGER STATION
PHONE

DAY-USE AREA

BOG TRAIL LOOP

SITES 31-74

BOG

LITTLE RIVER

SITES 1-13

SITES 14-20

SITES 21-30

TO FERN CANYON TRAIL

TO LITTLE RIVER INN

VAN DAMME STATE PARK

group camp where the forest meets the wetland. Watch out, the boardwalks are slippery when wet!

The two campgrounds, Highland Meadow and Lower Campground, are only a few hundred yards apart. Between the two, I prefer Highland Meadow, because it gets you up into the sun. Lower Campground tends to be dark and cool and gets the bicycle and foot traffic heading up Fern Canyon. Still, in the winter, it is the only campground open.

Be sure to reserve a campsite, especially for summer weekends. This coast is very popular. The beach is across busy CA 1, so be careful crossing—extra careful if you have children.

GETTING THERE

From Mendocino, drive 3 miles south on CA 1 to the Van Damme Park entrance on the left.

GPS COORDINATES

UTM Zone (WGS84) 10S

Easting 0435268

Northing 4346523

Latitude N 39° 15' 56.2753"

Longtitude W 123° 45' 1.3068"

20
WOODSIDE AND GERSTLE COVE CAMPGROUNDS

> *Sometimes in a campground, like in life, it's the little things that make all the difference.*

SALT **POINT'S CAMPGROUNDS** are a dream: impeccably clean, intelligently constructed, and full of details that show how much staff care about the park. These campgrounds are packed with little bonuses—water spigots painted to look like mushrooms, information boards with snippets about the natural life in and around the park, and fantastically clean, well-maintained sites and restrooms.

Situated on the rugged and beautiful Sonoma County coast, the park features more than 6 miles of coastline and 20 miles of hiking trails that wander through forest and grassy bluffs. The coastline here is a popular destination for abalone harvesting and features a protected underwater reserve where you can dive (no collecting). Trails depart from the campgrounds and lead about a mile (or less) to the beach. The two most popular hiking trails are the out-and-back coastal path from Salt Point to Stump Beach, and the loop through the pygmy forest. This pygmy forest, like others found along the coast, features dwarfed vegetation, and although the plants may look like they are struggling to survive, many of these shrubs and trees are more than 100 years old.

If you want more hiking, it's a short drive from the campground to the Kruse Rhododendron Preserve, where the main attraction are the park's namesake shrubs. They put forth gorgeous pink flowers in April and May. A fire swept through the woods on the south side of Salt Point State Park in 1994, and for years the hillsides were charred and nearly denuded. Ten years later, young pines are reinvigorating hillsides and the fire seems a distant memory; still, it's a good reminder to practice fire safety.

There are two campgrounds at Salt Point State Park, separated by a short stretch of CA 1: Gerstle Cove, on the west (ocean) side, and Woodside, on the

RATINGS

Beauty: ✿ ✿ ✿ ✿ ✿
Site Privacy: ✿ ✿ ✿ ✿
Spaciousness: ✿ ✿ ✿ ✿
Quiet: ✿ ✿ ✿ ✿
Security: ✿ ✿ ✿ ✿
Cleanliness: ✿ ✿ ✿ ✿ ✿

east side. Gerstle is set on a bluff above the ocean, and the sites are generously spaced, but since there are just a few trees and hardly any other vegetation, privacy is slight. Our first reaction to Gerstle Cove was, "We love what they *haven't* done to the place." The sites blend into the beautiful natural setting of coastal grassland, with several downed trees that have been left where they fell. A few sites at the end of the loop are too close to CA 1 for our comfort, but sites 9 through 13 are prime, where the sound of the ocean will lull you to sleep. From the Gerstle Cove campground, it's just 0.2 miles to the ocean on a trail. If your arrival at Gerstle Cove is greeted by strong afternoon breezes, you're in for a windy night with little to buffer the gusts—consider Woodside, instead, which is calmer.

The Woodside campground is comprised of two similarly sized loops: from the entrance station, lower Woodside is the first campground off the park road; upper Woodside is farther back and slightly uphill. After we settled in to our lower Woodside campsite, we walked the campground loop a few times. Honestly, we would have been pleased with any of these sites—there's not a stinker in the bunch. All of Woodside's sites are well spaced, with plenty of vegetation screening views out of the campground. In Upper Woodside, a few sites in the middle of the loop are open and grassy, but the rest of both campgrounds is dominated by bishop pine, Douglas fir, cypress, madrone, and a few redwoods. Ferns, huckleberry, and salal make up the understory. In spring, look for iris, golden violets, and labrador tea in bloom. In addition to ravens and Steller's jays (who will steal food left out in the blink of an eye), birds are plentiful, and we enjoyed waking up to the sounds of bird song. "Go light" solitude seekers take note: in addition to the park's car-camping sites, there are 20 hike-in sites that are the quietest of all. These sites are 0.3 miles down a fire road or trail, and most are well shaded by a dense redwood forest.

The weather along the coast is variable, but the general pattern is wet in winter, breezy in spring, alternately sunny and foggy in summer, and cool, calm, and clear in autumn. Reservations are recommended

KEY INFORMATION

ADDRESS: Salt Point State Park
25050 CA 1
Jenner, CA 95450

OPERATED BY: California State Parks

INFORMATION: (707) 847-3221;
www.parks.ca.gov

OPEN: Woodside: March 15–November 30; Gerstle Cove: year-round

SITES: Woodside: 79 sites for tents or RVs, 20 walk-in tent sites; Gerstle: 30 sites for tents or RVs; 10 hiker/biker sites; 1 group site

EACH SITE HAS: Fire ring, picnic table, food locker

ASSIGNMENT: Online or by phone; assigned by ranger; walk-in sites are first come, first serve

REGISTRATION: At campground entrances; reservations by phone (800)444-PARK; or online at www.reserve america.com

FACILITIES: Drinking water, flush toilets, firewood, wheelchair-accessible sites

PARKING: At individual site

FEE: $25, $6 each additional vehicle

ELEVATION: About 300–400 feet

RESTRICTIONS: *Pets:* On leash
Fires: In fire rings
Other: Quiet hours strictly enforced 10 p.m.–8 a.m; reservations recommended for summer weekends and holidays

MAP

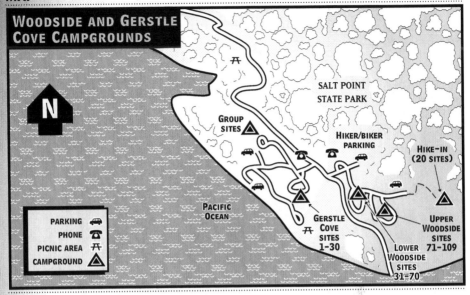

WOODSIDE AND GERSTLE COVE CAMPGROUNDS

SALT POINT STATE PARK

GROUP SITES

HIKER/BIKER PARKING

HIKE-IN (20 SITES)

PACIFIC OCEAN

GERSTLE COVE SITES 1-30

UPPER WOODSIDE SITES 71-109

LOWER WOODSIDE SITES 31-70

PARKING
PHONE
PICNIC AREA
CAMPGROUND

GETTING THERE

From US 101 north of Santa Rosa in Sonoma County, exit on River Road. Drive west on River Road 27 miles, to the junction with CA 1. Turn right and drive north about 20 slow miles to the park. You'll reach the turn for Woodside Campground first, on the right; the turnoff for Gerstle Cove Campground is just 0.2 miles farther north, on the left.

GPS COORDINATES

Woodside
UTM Zone (WGS84) 10S
Easting 0472075
Northing 4269020
Latitude N 38° 34' 9.0983"
Longtitude W 123° 19' 13.9979"

from mid-March to Halloween, but often the campgrounds are lightly used during weeknights. From our site, we watched the tall, thin bishop pines swaying in the wind, and chipmunks scampering about. Heeding the posted warnings about raccoons, we stored our food securely, and although we never saw them, telltale muddy prints on the locked food container in the morning were evidence that our precautions were wise. If you camp at Salt Point in early winter, scan the seas for gray whales migrating south to breeding grounds in Mexico. Lucky watchers might see whales breeching, but you are more likely to see a few spouts as the whales move through. In spring the whales return to Alaska with their calves.

You can get gas and pick up supplies at the quaint general store at Stewarts Point (8 miles north of the park), or from a few small stores along CA 1 between the park and Jenner. These stores stock ice, firewood, snacks, and beverages, but there are no full-service supermarkets in the area. Bring fresh bread, meat, or vegetables from your favorite outlet before you leave home.

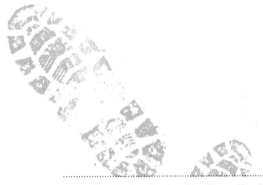

THE CASCADE **RANGE**

21
ASPEN GROVE AND MERRILL CAMPGROUNDS

EAGLE **L**AKE **IS SO UNIQUELY** beautiful that you have to go there, and it is so far from anywhere that you have to stay for a while. Don't bother lugging food supplies all the way to Eagle Lake—buy everything in nearby downtown Susanville, a town so western that you'll expect Wyatt Earp to saunter out of one of the square brick buildings on Main Street in his bowler hat, toting a six-gun. Then you'll look around and see the supermarket, gas station, and bank. All the same, Susanville is a real cowboy town.

There are two ways into Eagle Lake from Susanville. One is up A1 off CA 44, and the other is up Merrillville Road off CA 139. Both routes take you through a pass where you'll see Eagle Lake below—the second-largest natural freshwater lake in California (Lake Tahoe is split by a state boundary). All the campgrounds are down on the south end of the lake— all connected by a great bicycle path that winds its way through the woods and lakeshore. What a beautiful place!

The campgrounds—Aspen, Eagle, Merrill, and Christie—are run by the University Foundation, California State University at Chico, to give students majoring in recreation and parks management some hands-on experience. It really shows. The whole camping experience at Eagle Lake feels clean, intelligent, and supremely enjoyable.

Aspen Campground, for tent camping only, is a pretty little place on a knoll near the swimming beach and the marina. There's a store with showers, a Laundromat, and bicycles to rent. Eagle Campground is nearby, maybe a quarter of a mile from the marina, but too near the road to suit me. The last time I was at the lake, we camped down at Merrill Campground, which is for RVs and tents together. Merrill became my wife's favorite campground in California. Why?

> *True destination campgrounds—you have to work to get there, and you'll want to stay for at least a week.*

RATINGS

Beauty: ✰ ✰ ✰ ✰ ✰
Privacy: ✰ ✰ ✰ ✰ ✰
Spaciousness: ✰ ✰ ✰ ✰ ✰
Quiet: ✰ ✰ ✰ ✰
Security: ✰ ✰ ✰ ✰ ✰
Cleanliness: ✰ ✰ ✰ ✰ ✰

ADDRESS: Aspen Grove and Merrill Campgrounds Lassen National Forest Eagle Lake Ranger District 477-050 Eagle Lake Road Susanville, CA 96130

OPERATED BY: U.S. Forest Service

INFORMATION: (530) 257-2141, (530) 825-3454 (marina); www.fs.fed.us/r5/lassen

OPEN: May–October (depending on road and weather conditions)

SITES: Aspen has 26 sites; Merrill has 173 sites

EACH SITE HAS: Picnic table, fire ring

ASSIGNMENT: Some sites require reservations; also walk-in sites

REGISTRATION: At entrance; reserve by phone, (877) 444-6777, or online, www.recreation.gov

FACILITIES: Water, flush toilets, wheelchair-accessible, some full hookups (Merrill)

PARKING: Near site at Aspen, at site at Merrill

FEE: $18 Aspen; $18–$33 Merrill; $7.50 non-refundable reservation fee

ELEVATION: 5,100 feet

RESTRICTIONS: *Pets:* On leash only (no pets on trails) *Fires:* In fireplace *Alcohol:* No restrictions *Vehicles:* No RVs at Aspen, RVs up to 32 feet at Merrill

She liked the osprey family ceaselessly swinging over the lake looking for fish. She liked the Canada geese and the white pelicans, and she spent hours trying to sight a bald eagle. (No luck this time.)

I agree with her. Merrill Campground is even better than Aspen Campground. For one thing, I liked being away from the marina. There was less boat and vehicle traffic. The campsites are all well spaced, and if you want more solitude, you can camp off the beach. If you want lakefront camping, remember to make a reservation. The best Merrill sites are 166, 168, 170, 172, 174, 176, 178, and 180. The only problem with these sites along the lake is the sun and the light reflected off the water. There is some cover, but bring shade—umbrellas that fit onto your beach chair, a shade tent, or a sombrero. Don't forget to bring along buckets of sunscreen to slop on your exposed limbs.

Of course, many sites are first come, first served. You can also camp in a reservable site if you arrive and find it empty. Just check with the reservations host (in a separate trailer from the campground host), who will tell you if the site is open for the day. The best plan is to arrive, find a site that you would be happy with, park the car, then nose around to see if you can find something better.

Next, get out your fishing rod. The fishing is reputedly great. Although I did not personally wash a worm—and did hear some anglers grousing—Eagle Lake has a reputation for the famous Eagle Lake rainbow trout. Apparently, the lake water is alkaline, which gives this subspecies of trout an extraordinary flavor.

The Native Americans were always leery of Eagle Lake. Maybe it was the taste of the trout, or maybe it was the earthquake activity around Eagle Lake. But, in any case, they never established permanent camps around the lake. The Maidu and Paiutes would cruise through for a little fishing or hunting, but didn't stay long. They believed that a huge Loch Ness–style serpent lived in the lake. They also believed that Eagle Lake was connected to faraway Pyramid Lake by an underground river. Pyramid Lake is about 100 miles away in Nevada. What gives this legend credence is that contemporary scientists can't

MAP

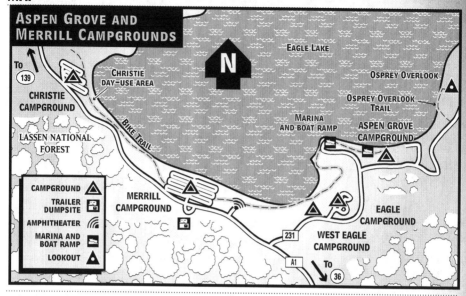

ASPEN GROVE AND MERRILL CAMPGROUNDS

EAGLE LAKE

To 139

CHRISTIE DAY-USE AREA

CHRISTIE CAMPGROUND

LASSEN NATIONAL FOREST

BIKE TRAIL

OSPREY OVERLOOK

OSPREY OVERLOOK TRAIL

MARINA AND BOAT RAMP

ASPEN GROVE CAMPGROUND

MERRILL CAMPGROUND

EAGLE CAMPGROUND

231

WEST EAGLE CAMPGROUND

A1 To 36

CAMPGROUND
TRAILER DUMPSITE
AMPHITHEATER
MARINA AND BOAT RAMP
LOOKOUT

seem to account for the apparently interdependent changing water levels in the two lakes.

For the two nights we were in Merrill Campground, we rented a boat (reasonably priced), tossed in sleeping bags and flashlights, and rode north until we found a particularly pristine bit of shoreline on which to sleep. (The pines of the south give way to sagebrush and juniper as you go north.) In the morning, we zipped back to Merrill Campground in time for breakfast.

GETTING THERE

From Susanville, go 3 miles west on CA 36, then 16 miles north on A1 (Eagle Lake Road) to the lake. To reach Merrill Campground, continue left on Eagle Lake Road 1 mile or so. To reach Aspen, go right on Gallatin Road 1 mile or so past Eagle Campground.

GPS COORDINATES

Aspen Grove

UTM Zone (WGS84) 10T

Easting 0688739

Northing 4491824

Latitude N 40° 33' 20.4769"

Longtitude W 120° 46' 14.9160"

GPS COORDINATES

Merrill

UTM Zone (WGS84) 10T

Easting 0685583

Northing 4490925

Latitude N 40° 32' 53.9089"

Longtitude W 120° 48' 29.9663"

22
BOULDER CREEK AND LONE ROCK CAMPGROUNDS

Family campgrounds, where folks come to enjoy the summer and the lake.

THE DRIVE INTO **ANTELOPE LAKE** through Taylorsville and Genesee is heartbreakingly bucolic. The road winds along little Beaver Creek through a Norman Rockwellian rural America. There are green pastures with cows belly-deep in grass, small New England–style cottages, nearby weathered barns pushed over by the wind, willows down by the water, and tiny stores with creaking floorboards and 19th-century-style cash registers ornate as churches and as big as Yugos. You can buy ice and beer and cold cuts, and drive on, dreaming of a simpler past. Was it really simpler? I don't know, but the roll of the beautiful land certainly speaks to me.

Then you'll climb up along Beaver Creek to Antelope Lake and go left to the campgrounds. Boulder Creek and Lone Rock are basically the same campground. Lone Rock is down by the lake, and adjoining Boulder Creek Campground sits back on a ridge between Boulder Creek and an inlet of Antelope Lake.

Generally, everybody wants to be down on the water, so the campsites there at Lone Rock are called PLs, meaning priority lakeside sites. They cost more ($18) and can be reserved. As with most campgrounds, these sites by the lake are well used, designed for RVs (since RVers outnumber tent campers three to one), and are packed in together. Still, it's waterfront property. So to be by the lake, be sure to reserve—because there is a steady supply of anglers and retired folks with RVs or trailers who'll take these sites if you don't.

Remember, too, that the campers in this neck of the woods mostly come from Nevada. They come in big pickups with overpowered engines fit to tow a trailer and an aluminum boat, and still have power left over to run the air-conditioner cold enough to frost the brim of your Stetson. They're used to desert, so they want to be by the water, but if you camp by a Nevada

RATINGS

Beauty: ☆ ☆ ☆
Privacy: ☆ ☆ ☆ ☆
Spaciousness: ☆ ☆ ☆
Quiet: ☆ ☆
Security: ☆ ☆ ☆
Cleanliness: ☆ ☆ ☆ ☆

pickup, trailer, and boat, it's like tenting next to a scrap-metal lot.

So tent campers should best retreat from the water, to the ridge at Boulder Creek Campground. Here, camp under the pines on a thick bed of needles. The blue lake sparkles through the trees. Everything is clean and new in the summer, after shedding about 20 feet of winter snow. Only on big holiday weekends does Boulder Creek get much play, so don't plan on having too many neighbors.

However, there are birds: cormorants, mergansers, grebes, coots, killdeer, geese, and great blue herons. I saw signs of beaver and what looked like an osprey. An owl (probably a great horned owl) hooted at night. I hiked up a logging spur on the south side of the lake and saw mule deer. I visited the log cabin and gravesites, and the dam information site.

It seems that Antelope Lake was not always a lake. Before California's Department of Water Resources built the dam in 1964, this was a wet, fertile valley. Maidu Native Americans came from their villages down near Taylorsville and Genesee in the summer to fish, hunt, and dig camus tubers and cattail rhizomes. They peeled back the cattail root to its core and made flour from it. Early in the summer, they would steam the green-bloom cattail spikes to eat like corn on the cob. They would dry the cattail leaves and use these for weaving. The camus bulb was cooked in a stone-lined earth pit for 24 hours, then either eaten straightaway or dried in the sun for later consumption.

The advent of the forty-niners was the demise of the Maidu. Whites moved in, and the Antelope Lake area supplied the mining camps with forage, butter, and cheese. Visit the pioneer cabin and gravesites on the south side of the lake. Imagine what it was like for the folks living there. Only the lucky ones had log cabins with doors and windows. Most lived in tents or shacks with dirt floors and canvas ceilings. It was harsh. In fact, many people remembered the westward crossing more fondly than their life on the frontier. At least then they had traveling companions and dreams.

In the new land, before kerosene, there was no whale oil or tallow for candles. So the women used

KEY INFORMATION

ADDRESS: Boulder Creek and Lone Rock Campground Plumas National Forest Mt. Hough Ranger District 39696 Highway 70 Quincy, CA 95971

OPERATED BY: U.S. Forest Service; Northwest Park Management

INFORMATION: (530) 283-0555; www.fs.fed.us/r5/plumas; www.ucampwithus.com

OPEN: May–mid-October (weather permitting)

SITES: Boulder Creek has 70 sites for tents or RVs; Lone Rock has 86 sites for tents or RVs

EACH SITE HAS: Picnic table, fireplace, barbecue grill

ASSIGNMENT: First come, first served; reservations available

REGISTRATION: At entrance; reserve by phone, (877) 444-6777, or online, www.reserveusa.com

FACILITIES: Water, vault toilets, wheelchair-accessible sites

PARKING: At individual site

FEE: $20–$35 at Boulder; $20–$22 at Lone Rock; $9 nonrefundable reservation fee

ELEVATION: 5,000 feet

RESTRICTIONS: *Pets:* On leash only *Fires:* In fireplace *Alcohol:* No restrictions *Vehicles:* RVs up to 27 feet *Other:* 14-day stay limit; don't leave food out; put food in car trunk

MAP

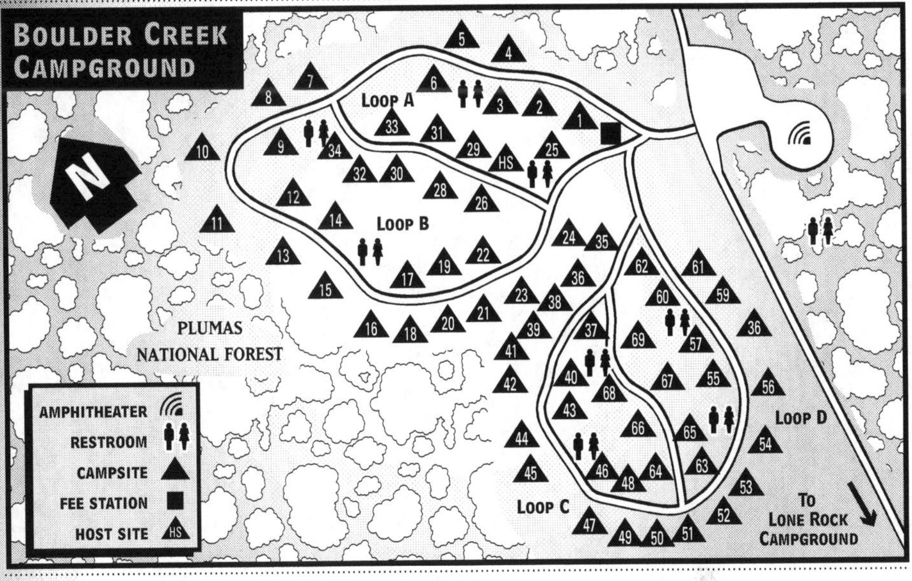
BOULDER CREEK CAMPGROUND
N
LOOP A
LOOP B
LOOP C
LOOP D
PLUMAS NATIONAL FOREST
TO LONE ROCK CAMPGROUND
AMPHITHEATER
RESTROOM
CAMPSITE
FEE STATION
HOST SITE
HS

GETTING THERE

From Taylorsville, take Beckwourth Genesee and Indian Creek Road (FS 172) northeast. Turn left at the dam, and go about 1 mile to the campgrounds.

deer tallow. They papered the walls of their shacks with newspapers and reread the articles as they lived there. With no jars to can wild fruit, the women cooked the fruit, dried it, and hung it like beef jerky. Some learned to make flour from roots and acorns, if they had the stomach for it. (Few did.) And, indeed, many of the forty-niners found themselves living with Native American women because they just "plain et better."

On the other hand, a forty-niner would ride 70 miles to pay $20 in gold dust just to take a fresh-cooked biscuit from the hand of a white woman in a dress. Such was the strength of the men's longing for their lives back home.

GPS COORDINATES

Boulder Creek

UTM Zone (WGS84) 10T

Easting 0703184

Northing 4451728

Latitude N 40° 11' 28.8707"

Longtitude W 120° 36' 47.2070"

MAP

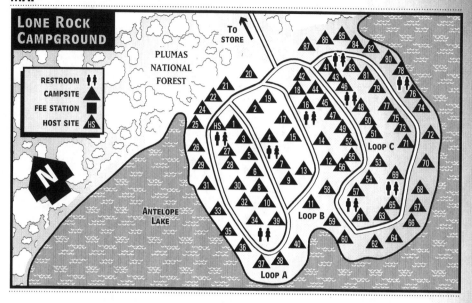

GPS COORDINATES

	Lone Rock
UTM Zone (WGS84)	10T
Easting	0702737
Northing	4452120
Latitude	N 40° 11' 41.9641"
Longtitude	W 120° 37' 5.6533"

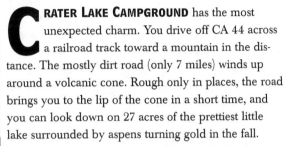

> *In the fall, when the aspens go gold, this little campground is pretty and fun.*

CRATER LAKE CAMPGROUND has the most unexpected charm. You drive off CA 44 across a railroad track toward a mountain in the distance. The mostly dirt road (only 7 miles) winds up around a volcanic cone. Rough only in places, the road brings you to the lip of the cone in a short time, and you can look down on 27 acres of the prettiest little lake surrounded by aspens turning gold in the fall.

This is a small campground—only 17 campsites, and most of them are pitched wrong or too small for even small RVs, so this is prime tent camping. The sites are sprinkled up and down the loop to the lake's edge. The last time I was there, in September, we camped right on the lakeshore—no one else was there. The aspens (*Populus tremuloides*) were turning orange, yellow, and red against the black volcanic rock of the crater. What a beautiful spot!

California's Crater Lake is part of the great lava plateau, including Lassen Volcanic National Park and Lava Beds National Monument in Northern California and, in Oregon, Crater Lake National Park (not *our* Crater Lake). Lassen Peak last erupted in May 1914 for a seven-year cycle of sporadic outbursts. When will it go off again? Soon, in geologic time, but nobody really knows for certain.

Part of Crater Lake Campground's charm is being out in the middle of nowhere. The nearest reliable food supply is Susanville, an authentic cowboy town, which manages to have a modern supermarket and cash machine at the Bank of America. Gas, beer, and ice can be had at Old Station, west on CA 44 at the junction of CA 89. But if you want fresh meat, only Susanville will do.

Fishing on Crater Lake is pretty good, especially after it is stocked—and the 94-foot-deep lake is host to

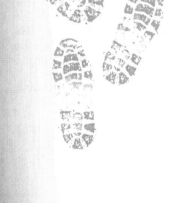

RATINGS

Beauty: ☆ ☆ ☆ ☆ ☆
Privacy: ☆ ☆ ☆ ☆
Spaciousness: ☆ ☆ ☆ ☆
Quiet: ☆ ☆ ☆ ☆ ☆
Security: ☆ ☆ ☆ ☆ ☆
Cleanliness: ☆ ☆ ☆ ☆

freshwater crawdads that in good years can be trapped for a one-crawdad, one-bite meal. A ranger I spoke to says the crawdad population goes up and down—in the 1980s the crawdads were especially prolific.

There is a hike around the lake. Back where the access road comes over the lip of the cone, there are several lumber roads heading out north. My wife and I walked all of them, then tried some cross-country trekking and found it easy. You can easily hike through the patches of pine down into Harvey Valley or Pine Creek Valley. Still, I think of Crater Lake Campground as a one-night stop at an impossibly beautiful spot or a place to springboard by car to other adventures (like all of Lassen Volcanic National Park).

There is a beguiling island out in the middle of the lake. To get there, you'll need a watercraft. A canoe or kayak will do fine, as will an inflatable craft of some sort. You can have lots of fun floating around the tiny lake, fishing or reading, or sunbathing on the island, with an occasional suicidally cold dip into the freezing water. On a nice day there is nothing better than the hot sun on your body and the feeling of the cold water through a few inches of insulating soft air compressed by the not-too-thick sides of your blow-up raft or kayak (buy the inexpensive electric pump that runs off your car's cigarette lighter).

Good hiking, biking, or horseback riding is found nearby, on the Bizz Johnson Trail along the Susan River and the old Fernley & Lassen Railroad route from Susanville to Duck Lake, 4 miles north of West-wood. The Lassen National Forest Information Station, at the intersection of Route 44 and the Crater Lake Campground (FS 32N08), will cheerfully give you the Bizz Johnson Trail brochure, along with information on where to access the trail and where to rent bicycles or horses in Susanville.

Find more good hiking in Lassen Volcanic National Park at the Butte Lake trailheads, just a short way from Crater Lake Campground. Go out to CA 44, then head west a few miles to FS 32N21. This road climbs 2.4 miles to Butte Creek Campground, then 4.1 miles to Butte Lake Ranger Station.

KEY INFORMATION

ADDRESS: Crater Lake Campground Lassen National Forest Eagle Lake Ranger District 477-050 Eagle Lake Road Susanville, CA 96130

OPERATED BY: U.S. Forest Service

INFORMATION: (530) 257-4188; www.fs.fed.us/r5/lassen

OPEN: June–October

SITES: 17 sites for tents or small campers

EACH SITE HAS: Picnic table, fireplace

ASSIGNMENT: First come, first served; no reservations accepted

REGISTRATION: By entrance

FACILITIES: Well water, vault toilets

PARKING: At individual site

FEE: $12

ELEVATION: 6,800 feet

RESTRICTIONS: *Pets:* On leash only
Fires: In fireplace
Alcohol: No restrictions
Vehicles: No trailers over 20 feet

MAP

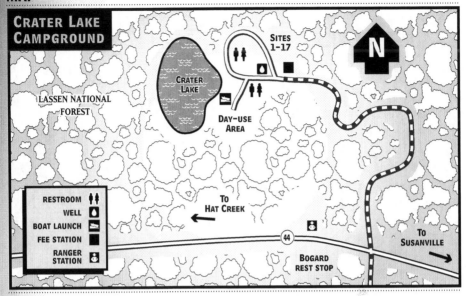

CRATER LAKE CAMPGROUND

SITES 1-17

LASSEN NATIONAL FOREST

CRATER LAKE

DAY-USE AREA

N

RESTROOM

WELL

BOAT LAUNCH

FEE STATION

RANGER STATION

TO HAT CREEK

44

BOGARD REST STOP

TO SUSANVILLE

GETTING THERE

From Susanville, head 28 miles west on CA 44 to the Lassen National Forest Information Center (and Bogard Work Center). Then drive north for 7 miles on FS 32N08 to the Crater Lake Campground. *Note:* The roads here are rather rough—take caution.

An easy hike from the north side of the Butte Lake parking lot is the trail to Bathtub Lake (warm, safe swimming). Climb about 500 yards and you'll see two small lakes. The northernmost one is Bathtub, and both lakes will do for swimming. There are other trails from this Butte Lake area (get information at the ranger station) for more ambitious hikers.

For another great expedition, take CA 44 east toward Susanville, then A1 north to Eagle Lake. Go right on Gallatin Road and find the beach and marina. A good boat with a motor runs about $50 per day, and you could spend a week fishing for the singular lake trout and exploring the miles of shore.

GPS COORDINATES

UTM Zone (WGS84) 10T

Easting 0665537

Northing 4499174

Latitude N 40° 37' 36.5772"

Longtitude W 121° 2' 33.9253"

HEMLOCK CAMPGROUND

LAST TIME MY WIFE AND I came into Hemlock Campground on Medicine Lake, all we could see were black clouds over the mountain, stretching off as far as Washington state, according to the radio weather reports. By the time we reached the lake, the tulle fog was blowing in, with rain not too far behind it. We got our tent up, our gear stowed, the flashlights turned on, and the travel Scrabble game set up before the rain turned to blinding sleet. It blew and blew, then the sleet turned to snow, and we put in earplugs so we wouldn't hear the flapping of the tent fly. After all that, then it was morning, the sun was blazing off blue Medicine Lake, and the fish were jumping.

Medicine Lake is beautiful. Hemlock Campground is the first of the three campgrounds you come to on the east side of the lake. After Hemlock you reach A. H. Hogue, then Medicine Lake. All three are fine campgrounds. Hemlock is more geared to tents, with fewer flat places to park RVs. A. H. Hogue is a little flatter, but still favors tents. Flat Medicine Lake Campground attracts the majority of the RVs and trailers.

Hemlock Campground is nearest the beach and boat launch. God knows how, but the beach is composed of actual white sand. It even has a natural kiddie pool, protected by a sandbar. Medicine Lake does allow motorboats, but felicitously, water-skiers are only permitted on the lake between 10 a.m. and 4 p.m. This leaves anglers free to troll in the morning and evening for the more than 100,000 brook trout stocked in the lake every year.

As we found out the hard way, the Modoc plateau has a mercurial nature. Its climate is "dry continental," meaning nasty. The weather can change between freezing and sweltering in a whisker. In August titanic thunderstorms on the horizon bring

> *A beautiful place to stay in the summer to fish and swim, and to enjoy nearby Lava Beds National Monument.*

RATINGS

Beauty: ✿ ✿ ✿ ✿ ✿
Privacy: ✿ ✿ ✿ ✿ ✿
Spaciousness: ✿ ✿ ✿ ✿ ✿
Quiet: ✿ ✿ ✿ ✿
Security: ✿ ✿ ✿ ✿
Cleanliness: ✿ ✿ ✿ ✿

ADDRESS: Hemlock
Campground
Modoc National
Forest
Doublehead Ranger
District
P.O. Box 369
Tulelake, CA 96134

OPERATED BY: U.S. Forest Service

INFORMATION: (530) 667-2246,
(530) 233-5811;
www.fs.fed.us/r5/
modoc

OPEN: July–October
(depending on
road and weather
conditions)

SITES: 19 sites for tents or
small RVs

EACH SITE HAS: Picnic table,
fireplace

ASSIGNMENT: First come, first
served

REGISTRATION: At entrance

FACILITIES: Water, vault toilets

PARKING: At individual site

FEE: $7 per vehicle per
night

ELEVATION: 6,700 feet

RESTRICTIONS: *Pets:* On leash only
Fires: In fireplace
Alcohol: No
restrictions
Vehicles: RVs up to
22 feet
Other: Don't leave
food out; 14-day
stay limit

impressive lightning but little rain. In winter the wind blows bitter cold. Pack a bathing suit and a ski jacket. You never know what to expect up here.

This is an incredibly dramatic landscape. No wonder: Hemlock Campground sits atop a 100-square-mile volcano—more massive than Mount Shasta. You don't notice it because the Medicine Lake Highlands come on you as slowly as the curve of the sea. Go see Mammoth Crater north of Medicine Lake to look inside the belly of the beast. And Mammoth Crater is not even the mouth of the volcano, which is actually 6 miles south, near Medicine Lake.

Take a couple of hours and hike around Medicine Lake. Include a quick detour on the trail by the Medicine Lake Campground to see Little Medicine Lake. The road past the campgrounds goes halfway around the lake. After that, just follow the lake. You'll find great places to picnic. It's not a bad idea to bring some bad-weather gear, just in case. Those little pocket raincoats they sell in the camping stores can come in handy. Little more than a light garbage bag, they are welcome companions when the skies open up.

Glass Mountain is a fun place to visit, reached via a short hike. Turn right out of Hemlock Campground. Drive south to FS 97. Go left for 6 miles, passing the first sign for Glass Mountain. Take the second left on FS 43N99. There isn't any real trail—just hike around. Part of this place is privately owned, so mind the signs. What you find here is dacite (the gray-colored stuff) and rhyolitic obsidian (the sharp, shiny stuff). The Modocs came up here often to gather obsidian to make arrowheads, spearheads, and tools to use and trade with Native Americans from as far away as the coast.

Other great hikes await down in Lava Beds National Monument. You have to explore Captain Jack's Stronghold (get the Lava Beds National Monument brochure for the map to the park, and cough up a quarter for the "Captain Jack's Stronghold" Historical Trail brochure). Try to find out how Captain Jack retreated, and follow the trail. The Thomas Wright Trail (white man's folly) is another hour's hike, as well as the Schonchin Butte Trail (short but steep). The Whitney

MAP

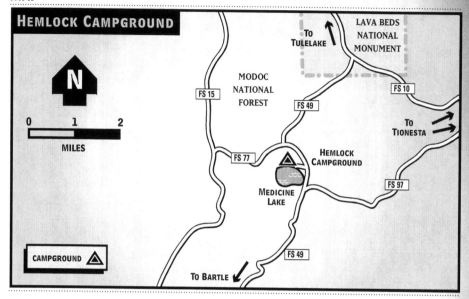

HEMLOCK CAMPGROUND

To TULELAKE

LAVA BEDS NATIONAL MONUMENT

MODOC NATIONAL FOREST

FS 15

FS 49

FS 10

To TIONESTA

FS 77

HEMLOCK CAMPGROUND

FS 97

MEDICINE LAKE

FS 49

CAMPGROUND

To BARTLE

0 1 2

MILES

Butte Trail is a day trip, so bring lunch and enjoy yourself. You'll end up on the edge of Callahan Lava Flow. In 1969, skeptics accused NASA of filming the lunar landing there. See for yourself.

There are two ways to get to Lava Beds National Monument. Go north on FS 49, which is the bumpy way (17 miles). Or take FS 97 to FS 10 near Timber Mountain Store at Tionesta (36 miles)—the smoother way. They both take about the same time. It's best to take the corduroy road going downhill, then come back the long way and get gas, ice, and cold drinks at the store. The next nearest supplies are available at the supermarket in Tulelake.

GETTING THERE

From Bartle on CA 89, head northeast up Powder Hill Road (FS 49) to Medicine Lake Road. Then go left to the Hemlock Campground.

GPS COORDINATES

UTM Zone (WGS84) 10T

Easting 0617474

Northing 4604782

Latitude N 41° 35' 9.9565"

Longtitude W 121° 35' 26.3291"

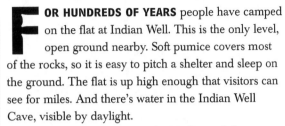

> *Indian Well is a true destination campground—this is the most awesome spot in Northern California!*

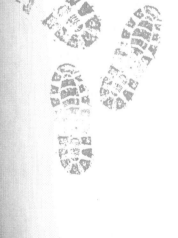

FOR HUNDREDS OF YEARS people have camped on the flat at Indian Well. This is the only level, open ground nearby. Soft pumice covers most of the rocks, so it is easy to pitch a shelter and sleep on the ground. The flat is up high enough that visitors can see for miles. And there's water in the Indian Well Cave, visible by daylight.

The first campers here, the Modoc and their ancestors, lived north of the lava beds along Tule and Lower Klamath lakes, subsisting on waterfowl, water-lily seeds, and fish, and cutting the tule reeds for bedding, hats, and canoes. In the fall, the Modoc camped at Indian Well on their way to the mountains to hunt bear, bighorn sheep, and pronghorn antelope, and to harvest manzanita, berries, and pine nuts. The Modoc were fierce and fought with the Pit River people and the Klamath to keep their rich lands. Then settlers came, and the Modoc fought hard against them and the U.S. Army. They lost—Modoc culture was eradicated to make way for ranchers.

Time has marched on, and many of the lakes from which the Modoc fished have been drained; the pronghorn herds are gone; and the bunchgrass the bighorn ate has given way to cheatgrass (an exotic plant from Asia). But we can still come here and camp, explore the Modoc's sacred lava-tube caves, hike among the sage and the rabbit bush blooming yellow in the fall, and imagine a time when this area was lit only by fire.

Lava Beds National Monument first shocks you, then rewards you. The land seems desolate and savage. The lava rocks cut like razors. Then you spot the vegetation and find that the land is rich and full of life. Here the continental plates were pulled apart, so magma rose up from the interior of the earth to form this land. There remain cinder cones, shield volcanoes,

RATINGS

Beauty: ☆ ☆ ☆ ☆ ☆
Privacy: ☆ ☆ ☆ ☆
Spaciousness: ☆ ☆ ☆
Quiet: ☆ ☆ ☆ ☆ ☆
Security: ☆ ☆ ☆ ☆ ☆
Cleanliness: ☆ ☆ ☆ ☆ ☆

strato-volcanoes, spatter cones, chimneys, Pahoehoe lava, and lava-flow caves.

I love Lava Beds National Monument. Of all my family's western trips when I was a child, I remember Lava Beds the best. Even as a little kid, I was awed by the elemental violence that created this land and how quickly the vegetation took over to give life. What an amazing place! From the campground, you can hike miles over the rock along Three Sisters Trail. Or drop down into any one of Lava Bed's caves with a flashlight and a map. The whole area is an incredible adventure, and visitors are expected to explore responsibly by themselves.

The visitor center is half a mile away from the campground, and there you can buy the Lava Beds Caves map book ($4.50). The Park Headquarters also lends flashlights if you need to supplement your own. Going into the caves is no joke. Bring warm clothes (cold air collects in the caves). A hard hat for your head is a good idea, but at least wear a cloth hat. Never go alone, and be sure to tell somebody responsible which cave you are going to explore and when you are going to get back. Gloves, knee pads, a first-aid kit, and food and water are musts if you go cave exploring whole hog—most people get bitten by cave exploration and can't stop.

Come prepared for hot and cold camping. Even in the summer, Lava Beds can be cold, and a stiff wind can make a cool day freezing. The dry continental climate of the Modoc Plateau is ferocious. The interiors of the lava caves are always cold. It can be very dry. Bring lip balm and moisturizing lotion. Bring a good hat with a drawstring to hold it on in the wind. Bring earplugs to use at night so that you won't lose any sleep listening to the tent flapping. Bring shorts and a T-shirt too, because with all the preparation for bad weather, the climate is bound to be balmy on occasion.

Food is unavailable at the visitor center. Buy real food at Tulelake (like a set from *The Last Picture Show*), which actually has a motel. Ice, beer, and hot dogs are available at rustic Tionesta (you have to go a few hundred yards off the road). Don't pass either town without getting gas—they have the only pumps for miles.

KEY INFORMATION

ADDRESS:	Indian Well Campground Lava Beds National Monument 1 Indian Well Headquarters Tulelake, CA 96134
OPERATED BY:	National Park Service
INFORMATION:	(530) 667-8100; www.nps.gov/labe
OPEN:	Year-round
SITES:	43
EACH SITE HAS:	Picnic table, fireplace, grill
ASSIGNMENT:	First come, first served; one group site takes reservations
REGISTRATION:	At entrance
FACILITIES:	Water and flush toilets
PARKING:	At individual site
FEE:	$5 per vehicle to enter Monument; or $10 7-day pass; $10 per night camping
ELEVATION:	4,200 feet
RESTRICTIONS:	*Pets:* On leash only *Fires:* In fireplace Alcohol: No restrictions *Vehicles:* RVs up to 30 feet *Other:* 14-day stay limit

MAP

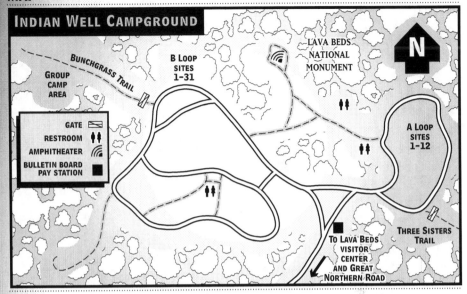

INDIAN WELL CAMPGROUND

BUNCHGRASS TRAIL

GROUP CAMP AREA

B LOOP SITES 1-31

LAVA BEDS NATIONAL MONUMENT

A LOOP SITES 1-12

GATE

RESTROOM

AMPHITHEATER

BULLETIN BOARD PAY STATION

THREE SISTERS TRAIL

TO LAVA BEDS VISITOR CENTER AND GREAT NORTHERN ROAD

GETTING THERE

From Tulelake, drive south on CA 139. Before Newell, go right on the Great Northern Road and drive 27 miles to the Lava Beds National Monument Visitor Center. The entrance to the Indian Well Campground is across from the visitor center.

Season permitting, try to camp up on the Medicine Lake Volcano, which blew off lava, gas, and cinders for a million years to give us the lava beds. In addition to three campgrounds, there's a good beach, decent fishing, and Mammoth Crater and Glass Mountain there.

GPS COORDINATES

UTM Zone (WGS84) 10T

Easting 0624061

Northing 4623438

Latitude N 41° 45' 11.0953"

Longtitude W 121° 30' 27.9830"

26
JUNIPER LAKE
CAMPGROUND

COME TO **LASSEN VOLCANIC** National Park and camp at Juniper Lake Campground because it offers the least crowded camping, hiking, and fishing in the park. Juniper Lake, blue and deep, is by Lassen Peak, Mount Harkness, and Saddle Mountain. Up until recently, in geologic time, Juniper Lake was not even a lake. About 200,000 years ago, all that was here was a depression with hundreds of feet of ice cap and icy fingers heading down into Warner Valley. The area warmed up, and a stream ran through the basin. Nearby volcanic Mount Harkness hadn't erupted, but when it did, it dammed up the south part of the basin, and—voilà!—Juniper Lake was born.

The last 8 miles into the Juniper Lake Campground are not great driving, but if you go slowly you can make it in any kind of vehicle. You just have to take your time and be careful. Plan on taking an hour to make that last 8 miles. Once you scale down your expectations, rough road traveling becomes enjoyable. Suddenly you can see the trees and the birds instead of a rushing green blur. Let about five pounds of air out of each tire if you want to stop your dentures from rattling. And remember, a nasty road is what keeps Juniper Lake from being a tourist hotspot. This is deliberate policy. Years ago, the Lassen Volcanic National Park decided not to stock its lakes and not to fix up its roads, hoping to staunch the stampede and keep the park as pristine as possible.

Do all your shopping in Chester before you drive into Juniper Lake, because you won't want to pop out for hot dog buns. Filtering water is lots of work as well—it takes a ton of pumping to filter out a quart of water.

Come prepared for any kind of weather. At any time, Juniper Lake can be either freezing or like

> *The most pristine campground in Lassen Volcanic National Park; but it is the hardest to get to, so come prepared.*

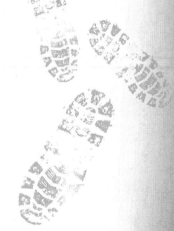

RATINGS

Beauty: ✿ ✿ ✿ ✿ ✿
Privacy: ✿ ✿ ✿ ✿
Spaciousness: ✿ ✿ ✿ ✿ ✿
Quiet: ✿ ✿ ✿ ✿ ✿
Security: ✿ ✿ ✿ ✿ ✿
Cleanliness: ✿ ✿ ✿ ✿ ✿

ADDRESS: Juniper Lake
Campground
Lassen Volcanic
National Park
Superintendent
P.O. Box 100
Mineral, CA
96063

OPERATED BY: National Park
Service

INFORMATION: (530) 595-4444;
www.nps.gov/lavo

OPEN: July 1–September 15
(weather permitting)

SITES: 18 sites for tents

EACH SITE HAS: Picnic table, fire
ring, bear box

ASSIGNMENT: First come, first
serve; no reserva-
tions accepted

REGISTRATION: By entrance

FACILITIES: Vault toilets

PARKING: At individual site

FEE: $10 park entrance
fee (good for
7 days);
$10 camping fee

ELEVATION: 6,792 feet

RESTRICTIONS: *Pets:* On leash only;
no pets on trails
Fires: In fire ring
Alcohol: No
restrictions
Vehicles: Small
campers only; no
RVs
Other: Check for
weather; use bear
boxes or other
approved contain-
ers; rough dirt road
not recommended
for trailers; no
water—bring your
own

August on the Riviera. Bring winter sleeping bags with a sheet—use the sheet over you and lie on the bag if it is hot. If it's cold, crawl into the warm sleeping bag.

Be sure to hike up to Crystal Lake. This hike is only about half a mile, but it's a killer. When you arrive, you'll need a swim regardless of the weather. Fortunately, Crystal Lake is warm! Why? I don't know. Juniper Lake is gelid. Maybe Crystal Lake is warm because it is on a south-facing slope. Bring a lunch and stay all day. Some say Crystal Lake has trout—I didn't see anyone catch anything, but folks were fishing.

The hike up Mount Harkness is another steep climb (about 4 miles round-trip). Catch the trail right from the campground. Hike up through the firs and pines until the woods open up into slopes of gray-rock lava from Mount Harkness. Keep hiking up until you hit the cinder cone, and then head west, up through hemlocks to the ridge. From there it's up another ten minutes to the fire lookout on the rim. From the lookout you can see just about the whole park. On the way back, a loop trail goes left and down to Juniper Lake. When you hit the lake, head east back to the campground. This loop is another mile or two longer than going back the way you came in.

Another good hike is around Juniper Lake, and this is more of a trek than one would expect. We underestimated the distance and forgot a lunch. The whole loop is about 6 miles, and there is enough up and down that we took three hard hours to complete the trail–cottage access road back to Juniper Lake Campground. There is a rocky point on the Mount Harkness end of the lake, where we went swimming in the cold water. After involuntary gasps of shock came welcome numbness, and then the exhilaration that keeps all those Nordic countries on their toes.

I heartily recommend bringing any rubber flota-tion device you can afford that will get your highly vul-nerable body onto the gorgeous blue lake but definitely out of the water. Think Big 5's Sevylor $50 blowups with an air pump powered by your vehicle's cigarette lighter. Never set your device down on sharp shale or pine needles—and come prepared with a repair kit.

MAP

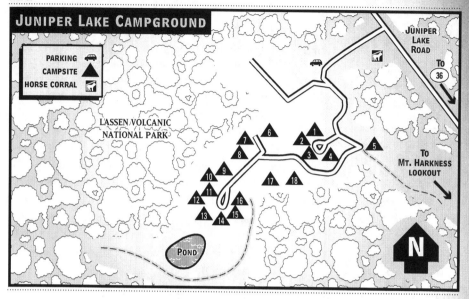

JUNIPER LAKE CAMPGROUND

JUNIPER LAKE ROAD

To 36

PARKING
CAMPSITE
HORSE CORRAL

LASSEN VOLCANIC
NATIONAL PARK

To MT. HARKNESS LOOKOUT

POND

N

GETTING THERE

From Chester on CA 36, turn on Warner Valley Road by the fire station. Drive 0.6 miles to the first junction. Turn right onto Juniper Lake Road and go 11 miles to the Juniper Lake Campground on your left.

GPS COORDINATES

UTM Zone (WGS84) 10T
Easting 0644613
Northing 4479233
Latitude N 40° 27' 4.2694"
Longtitude W 121° 17' 40.5708"

> *The queen of Northern California state campgrounds; Teddy Roosevelt called the nearby falls the "Eighth Wonder of the World."*

COME TO M**c**ARTHUR–B**URNEY** Falls Memorial State Park in the summer armed with reservations and children. You need reservations to get a campsite, and children to play with all the other kids teeming the campsites, hiking the trails, and cavorting on the beautiful beach by the marina. However, in the fall or spring, McArthur–Burney Falls offers peace and quiet. It is a premium state park with good swimming, fishing, and hiking, as well as comfortable camping with hot showers.

Lake Britton is a reservoir, but it is uniquely fed (design courtesy of Ma Nature) by an underground spring that fills the reservoir and keeps the 129-foot Burney Falls flowing. Teddy Roosevelt called the falls the "Eighth Wonder of the World." Back east in the Finger Lakes (upstate New York) we have falls like Burney all over the place, but we don't have black swifts building rare inland nests of lichens on the cliffs. Nor do we have water ouzels (*Cinclus mexicanus*) diving into the creek to walk along the bottom while feeding. The birds hold their wings partially open, and the current pressing on their wings helps hold them down. They can go as deep as 20 feet and stay down for a minute before shooting up into the sky like a rocket.

On Lake Britton, which has good fishing (rent canoes, paddleboats, and motorboats at the park marina), look for great blue herons, Canada geese, and a multitude of ducks and grebes. Bald eagles visit in the winter, when the weather gets too rough for them up in Canada. In the campground, we saw red-headed woodpeckers, evening grosbeaks, and a host of other birds. At night we heard the great horned owl, a creature with a five-feet wingspan capable of kidnapping a small dog. Yet the owl is constantly bullied by crows. How? Tough and clever, the crows attack together.

RATINGS

Beauty: ✪ ✪ ✪ ✪ ✪
Privacy: ✪ ✪ ✪
Spaciousness: ✪ ✪ ✪ ✪ ✪
Quiet: ✪ ✪ ✪
Security: ✪ ✪ ✪ ✪ ✪
Cleanliness: ✪ ✪ ✪ ✪

Around the campground you will find some good hikes—especially the popular Fall Creek Trail. This is a 1.2-mile self-guided interpretive loop that tours the creek canyon. Avoid this trail at all costs in the summer, except to access the trail that runs down the canyon to the beach on Lake Britton. At other times, this loop is astonishingly beautiful.

Another quick walk is up the Headwaters Trail to the underground spring and reservoir revered by the Ilmawi Native Americans living in nearby villages. The Ilmawi dug deep pits in deer trails to trap big game, so the first whites called the Ilmawi the Pit Indians. The underground spring and reservoir are the result of all the vulcanism in the area. Lava rock is all over the place, and sometimes water percolates through the lava rock and is trapped in underground rivers and reservoirs, or aquifers. One of these aquifers feeds Burney Creek and Burney Falls. Sometimes Burney Creek is dry for a half mile above the falls, but the falls flow year-round, fed by a subterranean source.

Good bicycling is found on the Old Highway Road that runs around the west side of Lake Britton (not CA 89). This road takes off from CA 89 about a half mile south of the McArthur–Burney Falls Memorial State Park entrance. It is a decent ride as far as the Cross Creek Lodge (a favorite hideout of Al Capone's), but then the road starts climbing earnestly up to CA 89. It's best to turn around at the lodge.

The lovely campsites at McArthur–Burney Falls were constructed by the Civilian Conservation Corps (CCC) in the 1930s. Many of them back into the canyon rim, where a trail heads down to the lake. With plenty of good pitch space, this is prime tent camping.

See how few bushes there are? At first I thought they were pruned by a busy ranger. Not so—a friendly ranger informed me that rainfall on the porous basalt rock quickly soaks too deep for the shallow roots of most bushes—another effect of vulcanism. She also gave me some good advice. When phoning for reservations, request a tent-trailer site. It seems there are 105 tent-trailer sites but only 23 tent sites, so your chances of getting a reservation are vastly improved.

KEY INFORMATION

ADDRESS:	McArthur–Burney Falls Memorial State Park 24898 CA 89 Burney, CA 96013
OPERATED BY:	California State Parks
INFORMATION:	(530) 335-2777; www.parks.ca.gov
OPEN:	Year-round
SITES:	23 for tents only; 105 for RVs up to 32 feet
EACH SITE HAS:	Picnic table, fireplace, food storage box
ASSIGNMENT:	First come, first served; reservations recommended
REGISTRATION:	By entrance; reserve by phone, (800) 444-7275, or online, www.reserve america.com
FACILITIES:	Wi-Fi service near visitor center, water, flush toilets, coin-operated showers, wood for sale, dump stations, 7 wheelchair-accessible sites
PARKING:	At individual site
FEE:	$20 ($15 off season); $7.50 nonrefundable reservation fee
ELEVATION:	2,800 feet
RESTRICTIONS:	*Pets:* Dogs allowed, on leash only *Fires:* In fireplace *Alcohol:* No restrictions *Vehicles:* 2 vehicles per site; $6 fee for extra vehicle *Other:* Memorial Day–Labor Day, reservations required; 14-day stay limit

MAP

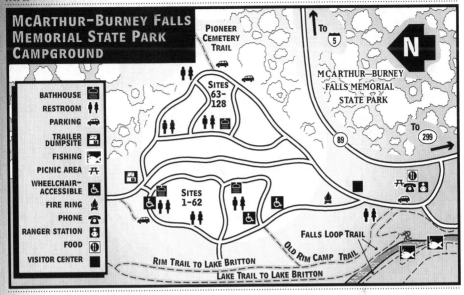

MCARTHUR–BURNEY FALLS MEMORIAL STATE PARK CAMPGROUND

PIONEER CEMETERY TRAIL

To 5

MCARTHUR–BURNEY FALLS MEMORIAL STATE PARK

To 299

To 89

SITES 63–128

SITES 1–62

BATHHOUSE	
RESTROOM	
PARKING	
TRAILER DUMPSITE	
FISHING	
PICNIC AREA	
WHEELCHAIR-ACCESSIBLE	
FIRE RING	
PHONE	
RANGER STATION	
FOOD	
VISITOR CENTER	

FALLS LOOP TRAIL

OLD RIM CAMP TRAIL

RIM TRAIL TO LAKE BRITTON

LAKE TRAIL TO LAKE BRITTON

GETTING THERE

From Burney, drive east on CA 299 until it intersects with CA 89. Drive north to the McArthur–Burney Falls Memorial State Park entrance.

GPS COORDINATES

UTM Zone (WGS84) 10T

Easting 0613298

Northing 4541702

Latitude N 41° 1' 7.1402"

Longtitude W 121° 39' 8.9426"

Upon arrival, you may ask the ranger to transfer to a tent site if one is available.

If popular McArthur–Burney Falls is full, camp at Northshore, a Pacific Gas & Electric campground just around the lake. This small lakeshore campground (30 sites and no reservations) always feels peaceful. Like most PG&E campgrounds, Northshore is clean, well run, and beautiful in an understated way. To reach Northshore, just turn left out of the main gate of McArthur–Burney Falls and drive north on CA 89 around the east shore of Lake Britton. Find Clarks Creek Road (otherwise known as Old Highway Road) on the left, drive 0.9 miles to the entrance on the left, and continue a mile down the winding road.

Lake Britton is enchanting. Mist purls down from the hills and spills over the water, and you'll expect a scene from a James Fenimore Cooper novel to materialize before your astonished eyes.

28
MILL CREEK FALLS AND BLUE LAKE CAMPGROUNDS

THESE TWO CAMPGROUNDS are out in the middle of nowhere—the South Warner Wilderness is tucked away in California's northeastern corner. It takes forever to get here, but the drive is stunningly beautiful and well worth the effort. Nowhere in the West do you find an area so pristine and so untrammeled. South Warner is big-sky country. There are real cowboys, real Native Americans, and real Thai food. Real Thai food? You bet, partner!

As fraternal twins often are, Mill Creek Falls and Blue Lake campgrounds are like day and night. Blue Lake Campground is big and bustling, with a boat launch and plenty of anglers. However, the well-designed campground—like a tiered wedding cake on a high point going out into Blue Lake—gives the campsites a private, secluded feeling. You are separated from your neighbors, and everywhere you look, there are the bright flashes of blue from natural Blue Lake. Come here if you have a boat and want to go fishing (5 mph speed limit).

I talked with some of the other campers and anglers. They had caught their limit of planted rainbow trout but talked about some big brown trout weighing 15 pounds. One old-timer said he hooked one earlier that summer and it towed him around the lake.

The only fly in the ointment was a helicopter we woke to in the morning. It seems that a lumber company is timbering the shores of Blue Lake and pulling the trees out by air. It was horrible. We packed up and left for Mill Creek Falls Campground.

Mill Creek Falls Campground is the best destination in the area for hikers and hiking anglers. A smaller campground, it features sites that are set in a hollow under the pines. It is clean and intimate. The smell of the woods is almost overwhelming. A short walk away (maybe a mile) is Clear Lake. A natural

> *Come to the pristine Warner Wilderness. A bit of a safari— this is the one trip you will never regret.*

RATINGS

Beauty: ☆ ☆ ☆ ☆ ☆
Privacy: ☆ ☆ ☆ ☆
Spaciousness: ☆ ☆ ☆ ☆ ☆
Quiet: ☆ ☆ ☆ ☆ ☆
Security: ☆ ☆ ☆ ☆ ☆
Cleanliness: ☆ ☆ ☆ ☆ ☆

ADDRESS: Mill Creek Falls
and Blue Lake
Campgrounds
Modoc National
Forest
Warner Mountain
Ranger District
P.O. Box 220
Cedarville, CA
96104

OPERATED BY: U.S. Forest Service

INFORMATION: (530) 279-6116,
(530) 233-5811;
www.fs.fed.us/r5/
modoc

OPEN: June–October or
first snow (phone
ahead for weather)

SITES: Mill Creek Falls has
19 sites; Blue Lake
has 48 sites, 19 with
RV hook-ups

EACH SITE HAS: Picnic table,
fireplace

ASSIGNMENT: First come, first
served; no
reservations

REGISTRATION: By entrance

FACILITIES: Water, vault toilets

PARKING: At individual site

FEE: $7 Blue Lake; $6
Mill Creek

ELEVATION: Blue Lake 6,000 feet;
Mill Creek 5,700 feet

RESTRICTIONS: *Pets:* On leash only
Fires: In fireplace
Alcohol: No
restrictions
Vehicles: RVs up to
32 feet
Other: Check for
weather and for
water availability

lake, formed by a landslide, Clear Lake has some big brown trout as well, though not in the same class as Blue Lake. But here you can enjoy solitude, the pines and rocks reflecting off the water, and the nice little jaunt to a place where you won't see or hear the internal combustion engine (although there is no guarantee the Forest Service won't let them cut around Mill Creek Falls—so write your congressperson!).

To reach Clear Lake, find the trailhead right across from campsite 10 by a parking area. There's a display map, but it's best to come equipped with your own South Warner Wilderness–Modoc National Forest map in case you opt to hike on past Clear Lake. With your fishing rod in your hand, head up the trail. You'll come to a sign pointing left to Mill Creek Falls. It's a 200-yard diversion to admire the falls. Back on the main trail, carry on to Clear Lake. A trail loop goes left around the lake. The beautiful lake is close enough to Mill Creek Falls Campground that you can hike up for a quick lunch, or even a sundowner, and still make it back to camp with the last light.

A great fishing hike heads up Mill Creek from the Soup Springs Trailhead. Drive out of Mill Creek Falls Campground and take a right on West Warner Road. Then take another right on FS 40N24 and find the Soup Springs Trailhead on your right. Hike up over a hill into Mill Creek Valley. Here you will hit Mill Creek and soon will see where it runs into Slide Creek Trail. Go left on the Mill Creek Trail, and head up the left side of Mill Creek for a couple of miles (the fishing here can be quite good). If you are truly ambitious and have the time, continue another 4 miles to the summit of Warren Peak.

The nearest supplies are available in the town of Likely, which has gas, ice, and other basic stuff at the corner store. But if you need meat or groceries, then head on up to Alturas. This place is hopping! Not only does Alturas have the county's only two traffic lights, a great museum filled with esoteric exhibits, the wild-and-woolly Niles Hotel on Main Street, and a supermarket on CA 299 coming into town, but it's also home to Nipas, a Thai/French/California–cuisine restaurant run by genuine Thai people. Nipas was

MAP

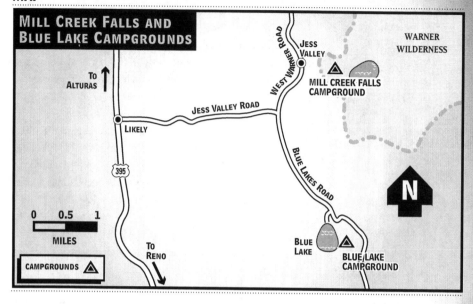

MILL CREEK FALLS AND BLUE LAKE CAMPGROUNDS

WEST WARNER ROAD

JESS VALLEY

WARNER WILDERNESS

MILL CREEK FALLS CAMPGROUND

To ALTURAS

JESS VALLEY ROAD

LIKELY

395

BLUE LAKES ROAD

N

0   0.5   1

MILES

To RENO

BLUE LAKE

BLUE LAKE CAMPGROUND

CAMPGROUNDS

mobbed when we arrived in town, by all the locals, as well as a blue-rinsed ladies' social group. It was wild (and delicious)!

GETTING THERE

Drive 17 miles south of Alturas on US 395 to Likely. Go left on Jess Valley Road for 9 miles to where the road forks. Go left at this fork for 2.5 miles, bear right, and go 2 miles to the Mill Creek Falls Campground. Go right at this fork and drive 7 miles on Blue Lake Road to another right turn. Go 2 miles here to Blue Lake Campground.

GPS COORDINATES

Blue Lake

UTM Zone (WGS84) 10T

Easting 0728014

Northing 4558399

Latitude N 41° 8' 41.5716"

Longtitude W 120° 16' 58.8180"

GPS COORDINATES

Mill Creek. Falls

UTM Zone (WGS84) 10T

Easting 0727927

Northing 4557748

Latitude N 41° 8' 20.5727"

Longtitude W 120° 17' 3.4151"

> *Read the camp register and become a believer—this campground is a jewel to cherish.*

WARNER VALLEY CAMPGROUND is a great place to visit. It caters to tent campers (the road in is not recommended for trailers), and there aren't even any bears (thanks to the new bear boxes). There is a ranger station a mile back down the road. There's the resort a few hundred yards up the road. The trails are spectacular. Hot Springs Creek gurgles by the campground, lulling the tent camper to sleep. The creek swimming is great. The sites are shaded but opened up, so you can get a sense of the land. Sites 1 through 6 are prime real estate by the creek, but the rest, on the other side of the road, offer privacy. The drinking water is cold and clean. Chester, with all the supplies a body could ever require, is a hop, skip, and a jump down the bucolic country road past little farms, old orchards, and rough little vacation homes. Good hikes splay out from the campground to just about everywhere. Or you can get in your car and explore Lassen Volcanic National Park, the most underused national park in the West.

Read the Warner Valley Campground register to see how revered it is: "Always come here, always will." "Dave's twentieth summer here." "Beautiful place to make a baby." "Trails are the best." "Lovely, quiet, serene." "Great swimming in Hot Springs Creek." "God's country." "Perfecto mundo." "Absolutely divine!" "Don't tell anyone about this place."

One minor disappointment is the fishing. Fishing is not great in Lassen Volcanic National Park. Since the mid-1970s the Park Service has not stocked most of the park's lakes and streams. However, near Warner Valley Campground, just outside the park, is some fine fishing. Try the Caribou Wilderness to the east—hike into the lakes. Caribou, Echo, and Silver lakes are well stocked, but folks can drive to them, so they get heavy

RATINGS

Beauty: ☆ ☆ ☆ ☆ ☆
Privacy: ☆ ☆ ☆ ☆ ☆
Spaciousness: ☆ ☆ ☆ ☆ ☆
Quiet: ☆ ☆ ☆ ☆
Security: ☆ ☆ ☆ ☆ ☆
Cleanliness: ☆ ☆ ☆ ☆

play. To the south are Lake Almanor and Deer Creek, both of which have great fishing.

Okay, so you can't live off the land at Warner Valley Campground. The only local food supply in the immediate area is the cook house at the Drakesbad Guest Ranch by the campground. They provide a Brotzeit (hiker's plate) to anybody who arrives at the cook shack clutching $6.95. For this you get a hungry-hiker trail kit containing selected slices of meat, cheese, and wine, beer, or soda.

Rooms at the resort run about $125 per person per night for three hots and a cot and a chair by the geothermally heated pool. Horseback riding on the resort herd is extra. Still, Drakesbad Guest Ranch is legendary and should be on the agenda of a "do everything" California explorer at least once in a lifetime. The place (settled by a relative of both Sir Francis Drake and the more contemporary Jim Drake of Santa Monica, inventor of the Windsurfer) is almost a century old. People come here the same week in summer year after year. So reserve ahead in the summer—call (530) 529-9820 for the brochure, or phone the long-distance operator and ask for the Drakesbad Toll Station #2 through Susanville, California.

A fun little hike from Warner Valley Campground is up to Boiling Springs Lake. The trailhead is on the left, a few hundred yards past the campground on the way to the visible Drakesbad Resort. Follow the obvious trail and cross Hot Springs Creek on the bridge. Reach a junction. A right takes you to Drakesbad Lake, Dream Lake, and Devils Kitchen. Go left and reach another junction, where the trail to the right goes to Drake Lake and, again, Devils Kitchen (another must-do hike, with fumaroles and mud pots). Follow the signs, and you will soon smell and hear Boiling Springs Lake before you arrive. The rotten-egg smell is the hydrogen sulfide from sulfur in the rising gases. The "bumping" sound is from the mud pots, which open and close like some monstrous earthen eye. Here's a hell even an atheist can believe in. The water is hot and yellow and green (green from some algae, and yellow from opal and iron oxide). It is hot enough

KEY INFORMATION

ADDRESS:	Warner Valley Campground Lassen Volcanic National Park Superintendent P.O. Box 100 Mineral, CA 96063-0100
OPERATED BY:	National Park Service
INFORMATION:	(530) 595-4444; www.nps.gov/lavo
OPEN:	Late May–October (weather permitting)
SITES:	18 sites for tents or small RVs
EACH SITE HAS:	Picnic table, fire ring, bear box
ASSIGNMENT:	First come, first served; no reservations
REGISTRATION:	At entrance
FACILITIES:	Water available mid-June–late September, vault toilets
PARKING:	At individual site
FEE:	$14 ($10 from early October to snow closure)
ELEVATION:	5,650 feet
RESTRICTIONS:	*Pets:* On leash only *Fires:* In fire ring *Alcohol:* No restrictions *Vehicles:* Not recommended for trailers or RVs *Other:* Don't leave food out; use bear boxes

MAP

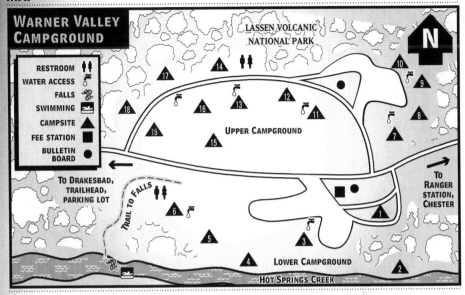

WARNER VALLEY CAMPGROUND

LASSEN VOLCANIC NATIONAL PARK

N

RESTROOM	👫
WATER ACCESS	🚰
FALLS	🏞
SWIMMING	🏊
CAMPSITE	▲
FEE STATION	■
BULLETIN BOARD	●

UPPER CAMPGROUND

TRAIL TO FALLS

To DRAKESBAD, TRAILHEAD, PARKING LOT

To RANGER STATION, CHESTER

LOWER CAMPGROUND

HOT SPRINGS CREEK

GETTING THERE

From Chester on CA 36, turn onto Warner Valley Road by the fire station. Bear left at the first junction (0.6 miles), and bear right at the next junction (5.5 miles). Drive 9.9 miles into the park and to Warner Valley Campground. (You will pass Warner Valley Ranger Station on the way.)

GPS COORDINATES

UTM Zone (WGS84) 10T

Easting 0636237

Northing 4478068

Latitude N 40° 26' 31.5958"

Longtitude W 121° 23' 36.9278"

to scald and kill you. Stay on the trail—you don't want to fall through the thin crust and land in an incipient mud pot.

The last time I was at Warner Valley Campground was in September, and we had the place to ourselves. I swam in the pool just below the wooden bridge crossing Hot Springs Creek at the beginning of the Boiling Springs Lake Trail. Other times, when the campground was busier, we went downstream and found great pools off the road below the ranger station.

Weather here can be dicey. Come prepared for both extremes, and do phone ahead in early summer to make sure the campground is open. The Lassen area is notorious for being snowed in through early summer.

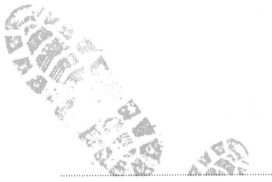

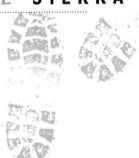

THE **SIERRA NEVADA**

30
BLUE LAKES
CAMPGROUNDS

HEAD UP **BLUE LAKES ROAD** near Carson Pass, but make certain you have all your ice and supplies, because it's a long way back to town. The nearest shopping is at Woodfords, or up over the pass and down at Caples Lake—but they don't have much. For the first 7 miles off CA 88 (Carson Pass National Scenic Byway), you'll breeze along the nicely paved Blue Lakes Road by the West Fork Carson River. Then the road turns to dirt for the last bone-jarring 5 miles to Lower Blue Lake. This poor old road gets washed out every spring, and the county has to go in and blade it up again. You'll pass lots of dusty guys in old-style Jeeps looking happy (there's some good off-road driving on Deer Valley Jeep Road, which cuts through the Mokolumne Wilderness to the Ebbetts Pass Road; and on the Summit City Road, which goes through to Red Lake on CA 88). All the scenery is spectacular. Then you'll come through the dust and pines and see the Blue Lakes.

The Blue Lakes have everything but motorboats: trout, granite islands you can swim to, meadows full of wildflowers, rugged granite ridges, and clear-blue water cold enough to ice down a six-pack. This is heaven.

I ogled Lower Blue Lake Campground and Middle Creek Campground, then inspected Upper Blue Lake Dam Campground, above the dam, before finally deciding to set up camp at Upper Blue Lake Campground. Why? I don't like to camp below a dam. This is earthquake country, after all.

One day in March 1872, at 2:30 a.m., a monster quake hit the Owens Valley. Felt as far east as Salt Lake City, as far north as Canada, and as far south as Mexico, it shook old John Muir over in Yosemite Valley. He wrote: "I was awakened by a tremendous earthquake, and though I had never enjoyed a storm of this sort, the strange thrilling motion could not be mistaken, and I

> *Come to Blue Lakes with a week's worth of ice and supplies because you won't want to go home.*

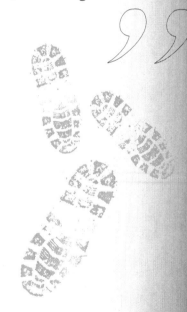

RATINGS

Beauty: ☆ ☆ ☆ ☆ ☆
Privacy: ☆ ☆ ☆ ☆ ☆
Spaciousness: ☆ ☆ ☆ ☆ ☆
Quiet: ☆ ☆ ☆ ☆ ☆
Security: ☆ ☆ ☆ ☆ ☆
Cleanliness: ☆ ☆ ☆ ☆

ADDRESS: Eldorado National Forest
100 Forni Road
Placerville, CA 95667, or
PG&E Corporate Real Estate/ Recreation
5555 Florin–Perkins Road, Room 100 Sacramento, CA 95836

OPERATED BY: U.S. Forest Service

INFORMATION: (916) 386-5164 (PG&E), (530) 622-5061 (Eldorado); www.fs.fed.us/r5/eldorado and www .pge.com/about/ environment/pge/ recreation/carson pass/index.shtml

OPEN: End of May– September (depending on road and weather conditions)

SITES: Upper Blue Lake has 32 sites; Upper Blue Lake Dam has 25; Lower Blue Lake has 16

EACH SITE HAS: Picnic table, fireplace

ASSIGNMENT: First come, first served; no reservations

REGISTRATION: At entrance

FACILITIES: Water every third site, vault toilets

PARKING: At individual site

FEE: $2–$24; additional charge for extra vehicles or pets

ELEVATION: 8,200 feet

RESTRICTIONS: *Pets:* On leash only
Fires: In fireplace
Alcohol: No restrictions
Vehicles: RVs and trailers up to 34 feet (difficult road)
Other: Don't leave food out

ran out of the cabin, both glad and frightened, shouting, 'A noble earthquake! A noble earthquake!' feeling sure I was going to learn something."

I want to learn something, but I don't want to get that wet. And, fortunately, both Upper Blue Lake Dam Campground and Upper Blue Lake Campground allay all the worries of the earthquake-conscious camper. Previously, we camped up at Upper Blue Lake Campground, figuring that the campground farthest from the dam was bound to be better. I think it still is, but recently Pacific Gas & Electric, which operates the camp, replaced the water system and had to cut a few trees and re-ditch for the plumbing.

I asked the hostess who came around for the campground fee where the good hiking trails were. She gave me "Bob's Hiking Map," which was a many-times Xeroxed godsend showing you where to expect the nude bathers, where to find all the little lakes, where to locate all the old trails, and where to find all the flowers. My family found flowers. There is a meadow just around the northwest side of Upper Blue Lake that was in spectacular bloom. We saw lupines, bachelor's buttons, forget-me-nots, shooting stars, buttercups, yellow snapdragons, swamp lilies, little pink button flowers, Virginia bluebells, penstamen, mule ears, fireweed, and more.

By the campground, the water is shallow and good for swimming. I hiked down through the dwarf mountain willow (deciduous and growing all over the place) and walked out into the water far enough to swim. Remember to bring shoes for wading. Even more great fun would be a cheap inflatable boat to loll about in, arms flung overboard, face to the warm sun.

People were pulling up fish all over the place. The best luck on Upper Blue was above the dam, from the shore. I saw people trolling the deep waters of Lower Blue where Middle Creek runs down from the dam. I heard somebody bragging about his catch up at Grouse Lake. A path heads to Grouse from a trailhead below Upper Blue Lake Dam.

It is also possible to access the Pacific Crest Trail. On your way in from CA 88, you will pass the trailhead before you get to Lower Blue Lake. You can

MAP

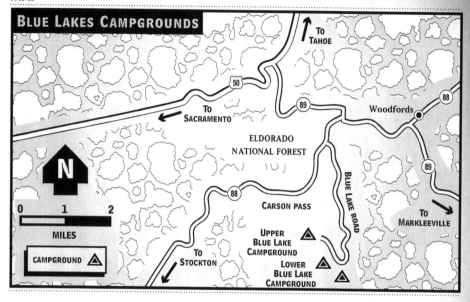

BLUE LAKES CAMPGROUNDS

TO TAHOE

TO SACRAMENTO

ELDORADO NATIONAL FOREST

Woodfords

CARSON PASS

TO STOCKTON

UPPER BLUE LAKE CAMPGROUND

LOWER BLUE LAKE CAMPGROUND

BLUE LAKE ROAD

TO MARKLEEVILLE

N

0   1   2
MILES

CAMPGROUND

go either way, although I hear the climb up toward Carson Pass is a bear. You can also access the trail by hiking up the Summit City Road above Upper Blue Lake Campground. Look for an off-road trail on the right that will take you up a ridge to Lost Lakes and the Pacific Crest Trail.

I loved Upper Blue Lake Campground. The pit toilets were immaculate. They even had those paper toilet covers, which really pleased my hygiene-conscious sister.

GETTING THERE

From Woodfords, take CA 88 west and turn left on Blue Lakes Road. Continue 12 miles (the last 5 miles are on a dirt road). First you will see Lower Blue Lake Campground, then Middle Creek, Upper Blue Lake Dam, and Upper Blue Lake campgrounds, respectively.

GPS COORDINATES

Upper Blue Lake	Middle Blue Lake	Lower Blue Lakes
UTM Zone (WGS84) 11S	UTM Zone (WGS84) 11S	UTM Zone (WGS84) 11S
Easting 0244151	Easting 0244334	Easting 0245236
Northing 4279776	Northing 4279433	Northing 4277548
Latitude N 38° 37' 46.6606"	Latitude N 38° 37' 35.7382"	Latitude N 38° 36' 35.5966"
Longtitude W 119° 56' 20.7889"	Longtitude W 119° 56' 12.7753"	Longtitude W 119° 55' 33.0382"

31
D. L. BLISS
STATE PARK
CAMPGROUNDS

Come armed with reservations, kids, water gear, a camera, and hiking boots—this is high-profile California camping.

LAKE TAHOE, THE QUEEN of California lakes, faces a mountain of woes—population and pollution threaten the lake's natural beauty—but if you come to D. L. Bliss State Park and hike down the Rubicon Trail toward Emerald Bay State Park, you'll see Tahoe almost as Mark Twain did. He wrote, "The air up there is very pure and fine, bracing and delicious. It is the same air the angels breathe. . . . The view was always fascinating, bewitching, entrancing." Tahoe still has the same effect, and D. L. Bliss State Park shows her off at her best.

Who was D. L. Bliss? Finding the answer took a bit of research. Finally, I tracked down Mr. Duane LeRoy Bliss. No nature lover, he was actually a ruthless lumberman who made a fortune cutting down most of the trees in the Tahoe Basin. After his demise, an heir guiltily donated some of the denuded acres to the state of California.

Now, besides being reforested and magically beautiful, D. L. Bliss State Park is a parent's delight. The place is crawling with kids playing under the pines and climbing the rounded boulders in the campground. We brought our big-city niece to Bliss, and within moments she was running around the campground playing hide-and-seek with all the kids. The flush toilets are immaculately clean, and the hot showers are heavenly after a day of swimming down at Lester Beach (the best beach in Tahoe for kids) and hiking the Rubicon Trail to Emerald Bay and back.

There are three campground areas. One area, campsites 141 through 168, is close to Lester Beach. These sites must be reserved. You must specifically request them, and they cost an extra $10 per night. The sites are packed in—tents only—and a little sandy, so it's not a bad idea to bring a tarp or strip of Astroturf to put in front of your tent, or better still, a basin

RATINGS

Beauty: ✪ ✪ ✪ ✪ ✪
Privacy: ✪ ✪ ✪
Spaciousness: ✪ ✪ ✪ ✪
Quiet: ✪ ✪ ✪
Security: ✪ ✪ ✪ ✪ ✪
Cleanliness: ✪ ✪ ✪ ✪ ✪

to fill with water so the kiddies can dip their feet before dragging sand into the tent, and ultimately into your sleeping bag.

The next group of campsites, sites 91 through 140, are a half-mile from Lester Beach. These sites are more spread out but still heavily used. I like camping still farther up the hill at sites 1 through 90 (site 22 is great!), where it is roomier and the ground is covered with a bed of pine needles. You're a mile from the beach here, but you can easily walk or drive down (folks camping can always park below even if the day-use parking lot is full). This is kid-o-rama as well, and has the advantage of not being on the main drag.

On the beach, the sand is white and clean and perfect for making sand castles. This is good news, since the water is freezing and fit only for walruses or Nordic rites of manhood. A couple handy items here are one of those cheap little blow-up boats and an electric pump that plugs into the car's cigarette lighter. With this outfit, you can float around the buoyed-off swimming area and read a novel. Or the kids can splash in and out of it and dump each other into the gelid water. There are no lifeguards, but people keep a pretty close eye on their kids and everyone else's.

Fishing at Lake Tahoe is either really great (when you score) or a total shutout. The clear, beautiful water is the problem. Fish need algae to support a food chain. Still, mackinaw trout, rainbow trout, and kokanee salmon can be found. They tend to stay at low depths in areas that provide them some cover—find mackinaws near Emerald Bay, in the northwest, and off the south shore. Rainbows lurk anywhere there's a rocky bottom. Nobody seemed to know where kokanee salmon hide. They just show up, and if you happen to be there— eureka! Everyone agrees the fishing is best in the early morning and evening, and on cloudy days.

The biking in D. L. Bliss State Park is poor since the park is on a fairly steep hill. Still, there is good biking around Lake Tahoe. One paved bike path leads to the Truckee River, a good ways down the northeast shore of the lake. Another begins below Emerald Bay State Park and curls around the south shore.

Hiking the Rubicon Trail is a must. You can access

KEY INFORMATION

ADDRESS:	D. L. Bliss State Park P.O. Box 266 Tahoma, CA 95733
OPERATED BY:	California State Parks
INFORMATION:	(530) 525-7277; www.parks.ca.gov
OPEN:	May–mid-September
SITES:	168 sites for tents or RVs under 16 feet
EACH SITE HAS:	Picnic table, fireplace, bear-proof lockers
ASSIGNMENT:	First come, first served; reservations recommended
REGISTRATION:	1 mile past entrance; reserve by phone, (800) 444-7275, or online, www.reserve america.com
FACILITIES:	Water, flush toilets, showers, wood for sale
PARKING:	At individual site
FEE:	$25 ($20 off season); $35 for lakeshore sites ($30 off season); $7.50 nonrefundable reservation fee
ELEVATION:	6,920 feet
RESTRICTIONS:	*Pets:* On leash only in park. Dogs not allowed on trails, beaches, or Viking-sholm area. *Fires:* In fireplace *Alcohol:* No restrictions *Vehicles:* RVs up to 15 feet for trailers and 18 feet for motor homes *Other:* Reservations required on holidays and summer weekends; 8-person maximum; keep food in lockers

MAP

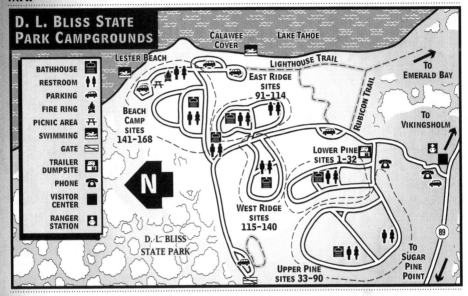

D. L. BLISS STATE PARK CAMPGROUNDS

LAKE TAHOE

CALAWEE COVER

LESTER BEACH

LIGHTHOUSE TRAIL

EAST RIDGE SITES 91–114

RUBICON TRAIL

To EMERALD BAY

To VIKINGSHOLM

BEACH CAMP SITES 141–168

LOWER PINE SITES 1–32

N

WEST RIDGE SITES 115–140

D. L. BLISS STATE PARK

UPPER PINE SITES 33–90

To SUGAR PINE POINT

89

Legend:
- BATHHOUSE
- RESTROOM
- PARKING
- FIRE RING
- PICNIC AREA
- SWIMMING
- GATE
- TRAILER DUMPSITE
- PHONE
- VISITOR CENTER
- RANGER STATION

GETTING THERE

From the intersection of CA 89 and US 50 in South Lake Tahoe, drive 11 miles north on CA 89 past the entrance to Emerald Bay State Park, to the D. L. Bliss State Park entrance on the right. Meeks Bay is a few miles north of the park entrance.

the trail (stop at the visitor center for a map) just south of Lester Beach or from a parking area just below the check-in station. Just cross the road and you'll see the sign for the trail.

Avoid Lake Tahoe's southeast corner unless you can bear 8 miles of motels and restaurants with outdoorsy-sounding names. CA 89 from the north or south is much friendlier. Shop in Tahoe City near the north end of the lake. A little store at Meeks Bay offers ice, beer, and sundries.

GPS COORDINATES

UTM Zone (WGS84) 10S

Easting 0748469

Northing 4319028

Latitude N 38° 59' 6.0503"

Longtitude W 120° 7' 53.1515"

FIRST OFF—QUAKING ASPEN Campground and Toiyabe Campground are just different loops in one campground in Grover Hot Springs State Park. Secondly, it is a family park. "Oh, my gosh!" the nice lady ranger exclaimed, taking a sideways look at my grizzled visage. "You don't want to be here in the summer when school's out. This place is full of kids!"

Well, if you have kids, Grover Hot Springs (named after Alvin M. Grover, one of the original Anglo owners) is the place to be. There are lots of other kids to play with your kids, so you can kick back for a change. There's a nice warm swimming pool watched over by healthy, young lifeguards; a nonthreatening stream full of fish and other interesting denizens; miles of trails up rounded hills; miles of nontrafficked roads to bike on; grassy meadows; a nearby western town with a museum, supplies, and horse rentals; a nature trail; hot showers; flush toilets; and a big, uncrowded camp to run around in like a wild animal.

The corollary to all the summer activity is that you must RESERVE, RESERVE, RESERVE! Make sure you have a campsite before dragging your kids all the way up here to find the place jammed. Some of the campsites here are by Hot Springs Creek. At first that might seem enviable, but this is where the fishermen fish and the excited kids play in the stream. Better to reserve a site off the creek, backed into the woods. Stay away from the bathrooms as well.

During the rest of the year, Grover Hot Springs is wide open for killjoy geezers who don't thrill to the trill of youthful voices. This is a beautiful park. It's well run and clean. The hike up to the waterfall is just enough to get the blood pumping without stressing the pacemaker. The hot springs bath adjacent to the pool is guaranteed rejuvenation with lingering powers.

> *Great for kids in the summer; good adult camping the rest of the year.*

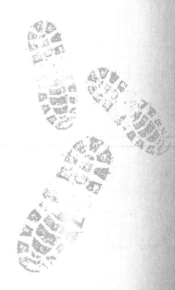

RATINGS

Beauty: ✫ ✫ ✫ ✫
Privacy: ✫ ✫ ✫
Spaciousness: ✫ ✫ ✫ ✫
Quiet: ✫ ✫ ✫
Security: ✫ ✫ ✫ ✫ ✫
Cleanliness: ✫ ✫ ✫ ✫

ADDRESS: Grover Hot Springs State Park
P.O. Box 188
Markleeville, CA 96120

OPERATED BY: California State Parks

INFORMATION: (530) 694-2248; grovers@gbis.com

OPEN: Year-round; closed Thanksgiving, Christmas, and New Year's

SITES: 76 total; 25 tent; 2 wheelchair-accessible; 49 for tents, RVs, or trailers

EACH SITE HAS: Picnic table, fireplace, bear box; water faucet every 3 sites

ASSIGNMENT: First come, first served; reservations recommended

REGISTRATION: By entrance; reserve by phone, (800) 444-7275, or online, www.reserve america.com

FACILITIES: Water, flush toilets, showers (except in the winter), wood for sale

PARKING: At individual site

FEE: $25 ($20 off season); $7.50 nonrefundable reservation fee

ELEVATION: 6,000 feet

RESTRICTIONS: *Pets:* On leash only
Fires: In fireplace
Alcohol: No restrictions
Vehicles: Trailers up to 24 feet
Other: Reservations recommended on holidays and summer; hot springs pool normally closed 2–3 weeks in September for annual maintenance; keep food in bear-proof lockers

The hot spring doesn't smell. Somehow, the waters issue forth from the earth without that rotten-egg sulfur smell. When the Sierra Nevada rose as one huge chunk millions of years ago, the violent changes caused faulting—that is, cracks in the massive rock structure. Water from the surface, then, works its way down through the faults to the magma where the rock is hot as hell, then boils back to the surface as hot spring waters replete with minerals it has dissolved along its way. The minerals include sodium chloride, sodium sulfate, sodium carbonate; calcium carbonate; magnesium carbonate; and a little iron, alumnia, and silica. This means lots of salt. I definitely felt better after my cure. The water is hot, about 103°F, which is cooler than the 148°F that it was when it left the ground. The hot pool is right next to the swimming pool.

There are good hikes around the camp. Find campsites 35 and 36, and you'll be at the extra vehicle parking lot where a marked trail heads west for the waterfall. It heads along beautiful meadows and through pine woods—mostly Jeffrey pines. Stick your nose right up to the bark and sniff. The Jeffrey pine smells just like vanilla. Another salient fact that I learned from the *Grover Hot Springs State Park Guide to the Park's Transitional Walk* concerns the Jeffrey pine's cones, which are primary food for the reddish-black Douglas squirrel. The guide asserts that "of the millions of seeds produced during the lifetime of a pine tree, only one, on the average, will grow into a new tree!"

On the trail to the falls, you'll cross some small springs and soon enough hear the falls. When the water is low, you can go up beside the streambed to the falls. In spring, however, count on climbing up the rocks just ahead of you to approach the falls. The round-trip should take you a little more than an hour.

Nearby Markleeville, population 100, is worth a trip. Visit the museum at the Alpine County Historical Complex. In 1861, Bactrain camels from Mongolia were brought here to be used as pack animals. Bad move. Conditions in the Gobi desert are a lot different from those in the Sierra Nevada. However, modern packers have made good use of the Peruvian llama, obviously better bred for life on the Pacific Rim.

MAP

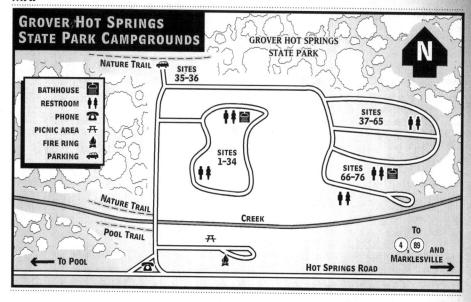

Another fun cultural trip is to Genoa for the Mormon Station Historical State Monument. This little park with its stockade, museum, and picnic facilities used to be a relief station for traveling pioneers. Basically, the tired travelers staggered into the station and were promptly overcharged for their bed, bath, and meal. Most men arrived on horseback and left on shank's mare. The owners of the station fattened up the horses and sold them back to new travelers for more cash. Right across the street stands the oldest tavern in Nevada, where the fleeced traveler could go to drown his sorrows.

GETTING THERE

From Markleeville, head about 4 miles west on Hot Springs Road.

GPS COORDINATES

UTM Zone (WGS84) 11S

Easting 0253499

Northing 4286807

Latitude N 38° 41' 44.0133"

Longtitude W 119° 50' 3.6162"

33
HASKINS VALLEY CAMPGROUND

> *This is easy summer camping, with lazy afternoons of reading novels and fishing on the lake.*

HERE'S ANOTHER BEAUTIFUL campground in Pacific Gas & Electric (PG&E) land. As usual, the campground is well conceived and well tended. PG&E is mindful of its image and sets out to curry favor with the public, ever apprehensive of its problems when it sometimes has to draw down the level of its reservoirs in late summer to satisfy us energy guzzlers in the flatland below. That's when folks look around and say, "Hey, Bucks Lake isn't a lake at all, but a reservoir contained by a dam. And Haskins Valley is named for the valley where the lake is now."

Still, I love Bucks Lake, Haskins Valley Campground, and electric lights, all in that order. The sites are set on a handsome pined knoll embraced by the lake. All you see is the waving green of the pines and the sparkling blue-green sky and water. What a spot to spend a week! This is kick-back-and-relax country. Quincy is just down the road, so you don't have to worry about serious supplies. There is a store right on the lake that sells sundries. In Meadow Valley below, the road splits to make a low road and a high road to Bucks Lake. Take the 2-mile-longer low option, Big Creek Road, if you don't trust your ancient automobile (and admire incredible dogwoods). At Bucks Lake, you'll find boats to rent, shoreline to explore, hikes to take, and a lake that warms up in summer to temperatures that suit the most spoiled swimmer.

Think summer camping. Bring a tent you can stand up in—and sit in your folding chair. Think about a screen house. There are voracious mosquitoes in this area. Out there when the bloodsuckers are buzzing in your ears, a screen house is worth its weight in gold. The last time I was out at Bucks Lake, I complained about the mosquitoes and heard the polite laughter of an elderly couple a campsite away who were sitting genteelly inside their screen house around a card table.

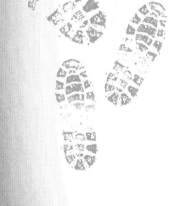

RATINGS

Beauty: ✫ ✫ ✫ ✫ ✫
Privacy: ✫ ✫ ✫
Spaciousness: ✫ ✫ ✫
Quiet: ✫ ✫ ✫
Security: ✫ ✫ ✫
Cleanliness: ✫ ✫ ✫ ✫

I found that Coleman sold a minimal version, and I bought it. Now I'm looking forward to sitting in it, reading a novel, and listening to unenlightened campers slapping skeeters.

Bucks Lake is heavy-duty cross-country-skiing territory. In fact, this area, notably Johnsville, takes credit for introducing the sport of skiing to the West. Apparently, miners from Norway and Sweden built "long boards" or "snowshoes" from planks up to 12 feet long, weighing about 20 pounds. Now we call them skis. The miners used them to get around in deep snow—for fun, they started downhill races above Eureka Lake. According to legend, they reached up to 80 mph; a long ski pole held between the legs was used as a brake or as a pivot around which to turn.

Quincy is a fun visit. Looking like a movie set for the all-American town, Quincy is the Plumas County seat and home to the Plumas County Museum, which chronicles Quincy's involvement with gold mining, logging, and the railroad. Imagine the wives arriving from the East to join their gold-miner husbands at Quincy. One wrote, "Our fare is very plain, consisting of meat and bread, bread and meat, now and then some rancid butter that was put up in the Land Of Goshen [the East] and sent on a six-month cruise by Cape Horn, for which we give the sum of $2 a pound." Of course, all this on top of crude log cabins, rowdy forty-niners, and the heartbreak of betting your all on striking it rich.

The museum also has a decent exhibit on the Maidu Indians, the previous leaseholders of the area that includes Plumas County (named for bird feathers a Spanish explorer observed in the river). The Maidu, who ironically never valued gold, did use gold-laced quartz for spear tips, knives, and mortars. They were low-key Native Americans who "trod very lightly" on the land, and at first gazed with curiosity at the forty-niners and their industrious ways. For a while, the Maidu were happy to find gold to trade with the white man for a shirt or a pair of pantaloons. Soon enough, however, the two groups collided, and the Maidu passed rapidly into history.

When you drive around Quincy, look at the

KEY INFORMATION

ADDRESS:	Haskins Valley Campground PG&E Corporate Real Estate/ Recreation 5555 Florin–Perkins Road Building 500 Sacramento, CA 95836
OPERATED BY:	Pacific Gas & Electric
INFORMATION:	(916) 386-5164
OPEN:	May 15– mid-October, weather permitting
SITES:	60 sites: 5 tent; 60 for tents, RVs, and trailers
EACH SITE HAS:	Picnic table, fireplace, barbecue
ASSIGNMENT:	First come, first served; no reservations
REGISTRATION:	At entrance
FACILITIES:	Water, vault toilets
PARKING:	At individual site
FEE:	$15
ELEVATION:	5,200 feet
RESTRICTIONS:	*Pets:* On leash only *Fires:* In fireplace *Alcohol* No restrictions *Vehicles:* RVs and trailers allowed (no hookups) *Other:* Don't leave food out

MAP

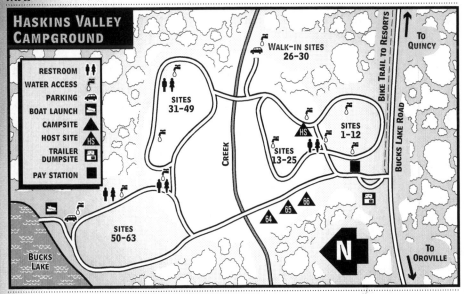

HASKINS VALLEY CAMPGROUND

RESTROOM	👥
WATER ACCESS	🚰
PARKING	🚗
BOAT LAUNCH	🚤
CAMPSITE	▲
HOST SITE	HS
TRAILER DUMPSITE	🚻
PAY STATION	⬛

WALK-IN SITES 26–30

SITES 31–49

SITES 1–12

SITES 13–25

CREEK

SITES 50–63

BUCKS LAKE

64 65 66

BIKE TRAIL TO RESORTS

BUCKS LAKE ROAD

To QUINCY

To OROVILLE

N

GETTING THERE

From Quincy, turn west on Bucks Lake Road, and drive 16.5 miles to the campground.

trees—the impressive oak, maple, and poplar. Quincy folks were loggers and they knew their trees. Look for the Morning Thunder Cafe—good breakfasts. Then drive up Bucks Lake Road—11 miles to the Bucks Summit Trailhead—and climb your calories off ascending the southern flank of Mount Pleasant.

GPS COORDINATES

UTM Zone (WGS84) 10S

Easting 0656159

Northing 4414968

Latitude N 39° 52' 13.4291"

Longtitude W 121° 10' 26.6773"

N 1852, **HUNGRY MINERS** needed red meat. And that's what Augustus T. Dowd was after, one fine spring day, as he chased a wounded bear up the Stanislaus River. Instead of lunch he found some of the biggest trees he'd ever seen. Using a string, he measured one of the trees. When he got back to town, the string was found to be more than 100 feet long. The story goes that nobody believed Augustus T. Dowd, and nobody would go with him to see the leviathan trees. Later, Dowd told everybody he had shot a huge bear, and when curious folks straggled after him to see the bear, they saw the Big Tree instead. Pointing to the immense trunk and lofty top, Dowd cried out, "Boys, do you now believe my big tree story? This is the large grizzly bear I wanted you to see. Do you still think it's a yarn?"

Indeed, the Big Tree is an awesome sight. John Muir noted, "The Big Tree is nature's forest masterpiece, and as far as I know, the greatest of living things. It belongs to an ancient stock, as its remains in old rocks show, and has a strange air of other days about it, a thoroughbred look inherited from the long ago—the auld lang syne of trees."

Hardly had the forty-niners' wonder faded when they resolved to cut a Big Tree down. They tried axes and saws—nothing doing. Finally they decided to drill with pump augurs through to the center from opposite sides. It took five men 22 days to accomplish the job. The tree fell with a crash heard from miles around. Immediately the bark was stripped off and sent to New York City to show the folks the wonders of California. And soon, folks came out to see the Big Trees.

They danced on dance floors made from the stumps. They rode horses through hollowed out Big Tree logs. They bowled on alleys made from the trees. They named the giants fancifully, as in "Pride of the

> *Open all year,
> Calaveras Big Trees
> State Park offers the
> best camping fall
> through spring.*

RATINGS

Beauty: ✿ ✿ ✿ ✿
Privacy: ✿ ✿ ✿
Spaciousness: ✿ ✿ ✿ ✿
Quiet: ✿ ✿ ✿
Security: ✿ ✿ ✿ ✿ ✿
Cleanliness: ✿ ✿ ✿ ✿ ✿

ADDRESS: Oak Hollow
Campground
1170 East CA 4
Arnold, CA 95223

OPERATED BY: California State
Parks

INFORMATION: (209) 795-2334;
www.parks.ca.gov

OPEN: Year-round for
limited grounds

SITES: 55 total; 22 tents; 18
for tents or RVs up
to 30 feet; 15 others

EACH SITE HAS: Picnic table, fire pit,
grate, camp stove

ASSIGNMENT: First come, first
served; reservations
recommended

REGISTRATION: By entrance; reserve
by phone, (800) 444-
7275, or online,
www.reserve
america.com

FACILITIES: Water, flush toilets,
showers, firewood
for sale; wheelchair-
accessible sites

PARKING: At individual site

FEE: $25 ($20 off-season);
$7.50 nonrefundable
reservation fee

ELEVATION: 4,800 feet

RESTRICTIONS: *Pets:* On leash only,
not allowed on trails
Fires: In fireplace
Alcohol: No
restrictions
Vehicles: RVs up to
30 feet, 2 vehicles
per site
Other: Reservations
recommended on
holidays and sum-
mer weekends; 15-
day stay limit; do not
feed bears; trees,
plants, and animals
protected in park

Forest," or after heroes, such as "Washington." They argued over what to call the Big Tree—"Vegetable Monster" was one name in vogue, briefly. But "Sequoia" seems to have won out in the end (*sequoia* after a Cherokee Indian, Sequoyah, who established an alphabet for the Cherokee language). Then they named the Big Tree Grove "Calaveras," after a skull found in some caves nearby—which was probably from an Indian burial.

Now we can camp under the Calaveras Big Trees at North Grove Campground—although the camping is lots better down at nearby Oak Hollow Campground. Never mind that Oak Hollow Campground has no Big Trees. It's a beautiful campground, and a good base camp from which to explore the Calaveras South Grove Natural Preserve. At South Grove you have to hike in like Augustus T. Dowd did, and earn your marvel by a sensationally lovely but untaxing hike. Drive to South Grove (or bicycle—good bicycling in the park!) and park. Cross pretty Beaver Creek—notice the tiny plaques nailed on the end of each bridge board, honoring a park supporter—and head off for the Big Trees.

The park offers a well-written guide for sale at the trailhead. It is an interpretive guide explaining what visitors see along the way. The last time I visited the South Grove, we double-timed out after seeing the Big Trees, and hiked up the fisherman trail alongside Beaver Creek until we found a good place to splash around.

The fishing was good too, as a strapping young lad proved by pulling two chunky trout from his creel for our inspection. He was wading around the creek barefooted and showed us his blue toes after he put away the fish. "Don't feel a thing," he cheerfully exclaimed.

Back at Oak Hollow Campground, my wife marveled at the clean, hot showers—quarter-metered, but 50 cents gets you a completely adequate washup. The campsites are nicely arranged, with enough space and brush between them so you don't feel crowded. Between campsites 123 and 124, a trail heads down to the river. Going the other way, you come to the scenic overlook.

Just down the road is Arnold. The supermarket is down past the golf course on the north side of the road. Before the golf course, on the south side of the road, is a

MAP

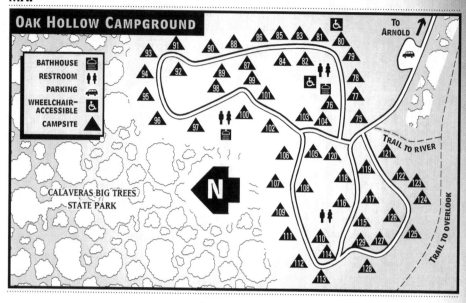

OAK HOLLOW CAMPGROUND

BATHHOUSE
RESTROOM
PARKING
WHEELCHAIR-
ACCESSIBLE
CAMPSITE

CALAVERAS BIG TREES
STATE PARK

To
ARNOLD

TRAIL TO RIVER

TRAIL TO OVERLOOK

sporting goods store where you can get fishing licenses, gear, and some friendly advice from the owner.

Don't forget to see Columbia State Historical Park. A huge hit with kids and adults, this restored gold-rush town offers gold panning, stagecoach rides, mine tours, and cold beer at the saloon.

It is worth it to make a reservation if possible. I always like to camp on the periphery of the campground so the backyard of the campsite is the woods. I also like to be as far away from the campground entrance and the bathrooms as possible. At Oak Hollow, sites 83, 85 and 86, 90 and 91, 93 through 96, 112 through 113, 123 and 125, and 128 are among the best.

GETTING THERE

From Angels Camp on CA 49, head 26 miles north on CA 4 through Arnold to Calaveras Big Trees State Park. Oak Hollow Campground is a few miles from the park entrance.

GPS COORDINATES

UTM Zone (WGS84) 10S

Easting 0736992

Northing 4239601

Latitude N 38° 16' 23.5596"

Longtitude W 120° 17' 27.0490"

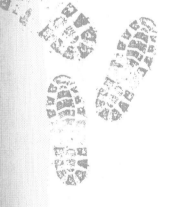

> *When the snow melts, Pine Marten Campground is heaven.*

PINE **M**ARTEN **C**AMPGROUND is on pretty Lake Alpine below Ebbetts Pass. It is popular, so try to come early on busy summer weekends to get a good site near the water. If you strike out, there are several other campgrounds within rifle shot where you can pitch your tent (there's a ranger station just west of Lake Alpine where you can inquire). It's best to come by Thursday and plan on staying a week. This is prime Sierra Nevada camping.

Ebbetts Pass, just east of Lake Alpine, was named for Major John Ebbetts, who crossed the Sierra Nevada here while looking for a route to build a railroad. He got the nominal credit, but he certainly wasn't the first man to cross here. For tens of thousands of years, Native Americans climbed the Sierra Nevada looking for cool weather and food. Their trails went to food sources and summering campgrounds. So, when the first gringos tried to follow their trails, they were often frustrated when they found themselves dead-ended at piñon forests and streamside flats.

Rightly, Ebbetts Pass should be named Jedediah Smith Pass, because Smith was the first European to make it over the Sierras, in 1827. It was rough going in the snow. "I started with two men, seven horses, and two mules, which I loaded with hay for horses and provisions for ourselves, and started on the 20th of May, and succeeded in crossing it in eight days, having lost only two horses and one mule. I found the snow on the top of the mountain from four to eight feet deep, but it was so consolidated by the heat of the sun that my horses only sank from half a foot to one foot deep." That's from a letter to William Clark—of Lewis and Clark—then Superintendent of Indian Affairs.

It snows heavily and frequently in this area. In July 1995, the snow drifted 30 feet deep at Pine

RATINGS

Beauty: ✿ ✿ ✿ ✿ ✿
Privacy: ✿ ✿ ✿ ✿ ✿
Spaciousness: ✿ ✿ ✿ ✿ ✿
Quiet: ✿ ✿ ✿ ✿
Security: ✿ ✿ ✿ ✿ ✿
Cleanliness: ✿ ✿ ✿

Marten Campground. Pacific storms sucked in through the Golden Gate head east to the Sierra Nevada below Ebbetts Pass. At about 7,000 feet, the clouds cool down and dump all their moisture as snow.

The last time I camped at Pine Marten Campground, in early June, I found snow drifts still there. Over the phone, the Forest Service told me the campground was open. I mentioned this to a Lake Alpine local who remarked, "Well, they don't see much driving around in their fancy pickup trucks, now do they?"

We parked our car in front of the first deep drift and carried our tent and gear into the campground, until we found a nice, level, fairly dry spot and pitched the tent. Our drinks went into a drift and I scoured dishes with snow.

A good hike out of Pine Marten Campground is to Inspiration Point. It gets steep in places, but you can get there and back in an hour or so. Pick up the trail just past the Pine Marten Campground entrance. There's a trailhead sign for Inspiration Point–Lakeshore Trail. Follow it through the lodgepoles until you start to climb. The slopes are steep and made of weird stuff called lahar, which was left by volcanic mudflows. The views are spectacular.

Up top, we sat down on a rock and ate a pound of sweet cherries we'd bought in the farmland below and gazed at Lake Alpine basin. It looked like a perfectly natural mountain lake. But looks are deceiving—Pacific Gas & Electric dammed up Silver Creek to make Lake Alpine.

The next day we went fishing in a rented boat but had no luck. I got a lecture from the previously mentioned local about how to affix my worm to the hook. He also asserted that using half a nightcrawler worked better than the whole worm.

It didn't matter anyway. Lake Alpine is gorgeous. There are islands of pines and gray rock—lots of trout for other people to catch, and warm rock to lie on while looking up at the clear cerulean sky. There are hot showers at the resort, as well as a great little bar and restaurant. Rent a boat and explore the shoreline. Hike up the mountains, come back, and jump into the water. It can't get any better than this.

ADDRESS: Pine Marten Campground Stanislaus National Forest Forest Supervisor 19777 Greenley Road Sonora, CA 95370

OPERATED BY: U.S. Forest Service

INFORMATION: (209) 532-3671, (209) 795-1381; www.fs.fed.us/r5/stanislaus

OPEN: June–October (depending on road and weather conditions); if gate is locked, the grounds are closed; opens after last snow

SITES: 32

EACH SITE HAS: Picnic table, fireplace, grill

ASSIGNMENT: First come, first served; no reservations

REGISTRATION: At entrance

FACILITIES: Water, flush and vault toilets

PARKING: At individual site

FEE: $20

ELEVATION: 7,300 feet

RESTRICTIONS: *Pets:* On leash only *Fires:* In fireplace *Alcohol:* No restrictions *Vehicles:* RVs up to 22 feet *Other:* Don't leave food out; 14-day stay limit

MAP

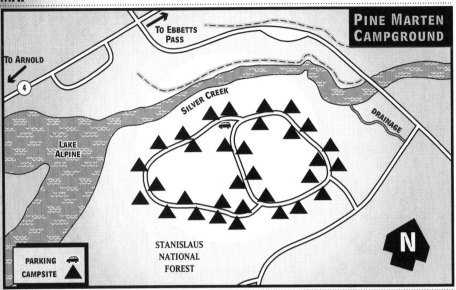

GETTING THERE

From Arnold, drive 29 miles north on CA 4, past Calaveras Big Trees State Park, to Lake Alpine (the town and lake) and the campground entrance on the right just past both of them.

GPS COORDINATES

UTM Zone (WGS84) 11S

Easting 0239215

Northing 4263424

Latitude N 38° 28' 51.7153"

Longtitude W 119° 59' 22.6718"

SARDINE LAKE AND SALMON CREEK CAMPGROUNDS

WONDERFUL **SALMON CREEK** trills past the Salmon Creek Campground, and Sardine Lake Campground is a mile away, just below the Sardine Lakes. Nestled into the still pristine Gold Lakes area, these campgrounds have it all: excellent fishing and hiking, fabulously beautiful scenery, and even a golf course. But come for the creek and the little lakes.

Scooped out of the flank of Sierra Buttes (elevation 8,587 feet), Lower and Upper Sardine Lakes are classic glacier tarns caused by the carving and scouring action of a glacier as it passed over bedrock. The low spots filled with water and became tarns. How beautiful! The Sardine Lakes are blue and clear and mirror the snow and rocks in the Sierra Buttes above. (Read John Muir's *The Mountains of California* for a rhapsodic description of the life of a tarn, in the chapter titled "The Glacier Lakes.")

No wonder the forty-niners fell in love with California, despite the wicked hand Lady Luck dealt them. Still, they remembered the beauty of California, and when Charles Nordoff (author of *California for Travelers and Settlers*) came through in 1872, he found that many of the forty-niners had stayed or returned to Gold Country to live out their days.

Every site at Sardine Lake Campground has a full view of the Sierra Buttes. The last time I was there, they were brushing out the campground, so we moved half a mile away to the Salmon Creek Campground, where our site backed up to the creek. Many of the sites there offer views of the mountains, but the rushing waters of Salmon Creek are equally scenic. The only slight catch in this otherwise fantastic campground is the road on the hill above the campground. From time to time, the muffler on a lumber truck overwhelms the splash of the creek, but this is a national forest, land of many uses.

> *These twin campgrounds show the best the Sierra Nevada has to offer.*

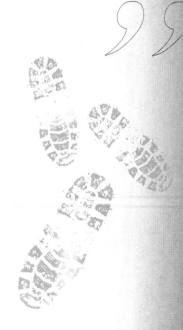

RATINGS

Beauty: ✿ ✿ ✿ ✿ ✿
Privacy: ✿ ✿ ✿ ✿
Spaciousness: ✿ ✿ ✿ ✿ ✿
Quiet: ✿ ✿ ✿ ✿
Security: ✿ ✿ ✿
Cleanliness: ✿ ✿ ✿

ADDRESS: Sardine Lake and
Salmon Creek
Campgrounds
Tahoe National
Forest
Forest Supervisor
631 Coyote Street
Nevada City, CA
95959
www.rs.fs.fed.us/
tahoe

OPERATED BY: U.S. Forest Service

INFORMATION: (530) 265-4531

OPEN: June–October
(depending on road
and weather
conditions)

SITES: Sardine Lake–29
sites (15 for trailers);
Salmon Creek–31
sites (7 for trailers)

EACH SITE HAS: Picnic table,
fireplace

ASSIGNMENT: First come, first
served; no
reservations

REGISTRATION: At entrance

FACILITIES: Water, vault toilets

PARKING: At individual site

FEE: $20

ELEVATION: 5,800 feet

RESTRICTIONS: *Pets:* On leash only
Fires: In fireplace
Alcohol: No
restrictions
Vehicles: RVs and
small trailers
allowed (no
hookups)
Other: Don't leave
food out

A few hundred yards up toward Sardine Lake is Sand Pond, which offers good swimming. It is round, a couple hundred yards across, and shallow enough for the light-sand bottom to pick up the sun. In early June, Sand Pond is warm enough to sit in the water in an aluminum chair with a book. Formed by a mining operation of the nearby All American Gold Mine, Sand Pond is prime for aquatic kids.

Early in the morning, Sardine Lake is besieged with anglers who troll slowly across the water (5 mph speed limit) before disappointment or triumph brings them in for lunch. Some of them stay in the neat cabins at the foot of the lake. I'm told the food in the lodge there is spectacular. I eyeballed the menu in the window, and it looked decidedly haute cuisine. We met an older gent fishing nearby, who told us he rents a cabin every summer on Sardine Lake.

He told us about the hummingbirds, too. It seems there are seven species of hummingbirds in Northern California, and six of them breed around Sardine Lake. I've actually seen and identified five of them: the rufous, the calliope, Anna's, the broad-tailed, and the black-chinned. They come iridescent green, blue, and red, beating their wings about 75 times per second, with their hearts pumping 500 times a minute. They are so quick and small you need binoculars to really take a measure of them. The prettiest is the smallest, the calliope, with exotic reddish throat whiskers. This little bird strengthens its nest with spider silk.

Later in the summer, good places to spot hummers are up by Donner Memorial State Park or down on the west shore of Lake Tahoe near D. L. Bliss State Park. Remember, if you don't see flowers, you won't see hummingbirds.

There's a fun little hike near the Sardine Lake Campground. Go toward Sand Pond, and you'll see the beginning of the Sand Pond Interpretive Trail. Immediately, the trail takes you through a "ghost" forest caused by some beavers who dammed up Salmon Creek and flooded the forest, killing all the lodgepole pines.

For lunch, do as we did—drive north on Gold Lake Road to the turnoff to Frazier Falls. The parking lot and trailhead is a mile or so down the dirt road.

MAP

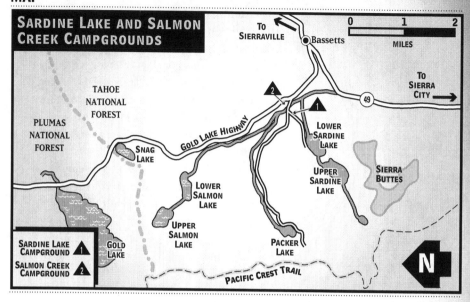

SARDINE LAKE AND SALMON CREEK CAMPGROUNDS

To SIERRAVILLE

Bassetts

0   1   2
MILES

TAHOE NATIONAL FOREST

PLUMAS NATIONAL FOREST

To SIERRA CITY

GOLD LAKE HIGHWAY

49

SNAG LAKE

LOWER SARDINE LAKE

LOWER SALMON LAKE

UPPER SARDINE LAKE

SIERRA BUTTES

UPPER SALMON LAKE

PACKER LAKE

GOLD LAKE

SARDINE LAKE CAMPGROUND 1

SALMON CREEK CAMPGROUND 2

PACIFIC CREST TRAIL

N

Take a stroll into the falls lookout, then backtrack to the granite rocks at the head of the falls. Picnic looking out over the mountains and valley.

For a great sunset, head for Upper Sardine Lake. There's an old logging trail that goes up the north side of Lower Sardine Lake. Hike up here about a mile, and—voilà!—there's another heartbreakingly beautiful but smaller tarn where you can watch the sun sink in the west, and praise the angel that brought you to the Sardine Lakes.

GETTING THERE

From Sierra City, go north on CA 49 about 5 miles to the junction with Gold Lake Highway. Go 2 miles north to the entrance to Sardine Lake Campground on your left. For Salmon Creek Campground, stay on Gold Lake Highway a few hundred yards more to the entrance on your left.

GPS COORDINATES

UTM Zone (WGS84) 10S

Easting 0704512

Northing 4388161

Latitude N 39° 37' 7.6621"

Longtitude W 120° 37' 2.7912"

> *Silver Creek
> Campground makes
> you feel the massive
> Sierra Nevada.*

CAMPING AT **SILVER CREEK** Campground is like sleeping on the shoulder of a huge beast: the Sierra Nevada, which is a huge hunk of granite thrust from the earth. It is tilted so the western slope is gradual, while the east side rises almost straight up. Silver Creek Campground hangs on like a flea just below the 8,730-foot Ebbetts Pass. The campground is on a piece of land like the prow of a ship, with the Ebbetts Pass Road running down the center. The north side of the campground has Silver Creek on its flank, the south side Noble Creek. The campsites are well engineered and clean—scoured by the winter and the dry desert air from below.

Native Americans came up both sides of the Sierra Nevada in the summer to escape the heat. It was easy to walk up over the pass and visit with folks from the other side. Yokuts from the west traded deer, antelope, and elk skins; baskets; acorns; and seashells for piñon nuts, red paint, strong bows backed with sinew, pumice stones, and obsidian from the Paiutes on the east.

The first white man to attempt the Sierra Nevada crossing was Jedediah Strong Smith. He came through California from the south with a band of trappers in 1826. Looking for beaver in the streams running down out of the Sierra Nevada, Smith noted "a great many Indians, mostly naked and destitute of arms, with the exception of bows and arrows, and what is very singular among Indians, they cut their hair to the length of three inches. They proved to be friendly. Their manner of living is on fish, roots, acorns, and grass."

Eager to get back to rendezvous at the Great Salt Lake, Smith and his men failed two attempts to cross going up the Kings River and the American River. Finally, Smith led his men up a Native American path along the Stanislaus River and over the mountains, near what is now called Ebbetts Pass. They arrived at

RATINGS

Beauty: ✿ ✿ ✿ ✿ ✿
Privacy: ✿ ✿
Spaciousness: ✿ ✿ ✿ ✿ ✿
Quiet: ✿ ✿
Security: ✿ ✿ ✿ ✿ ✿
Cleanliness: ✿ ✿ ✿ ✿

the Great Salt Lake with only one horse and a mule. They had eaten the rest of their livestock along the way.

At Silver Creek Campground, watch the stars move across the night sky and imagine you're on the deck of a huge ship—this hunk of granite that slides across the earth over the hot magma below. From time to time, a lone car's lights come down the pass. You'll feel the power of the mountains and sense the fear of the drivers, the inadequacy of their mechanical conveyances, and the coming snow, which will stop them all dead in their tracks. Old Jedediah Smith must have felt that way—awed, far from home, and scared to death.

A good day hike from camp is up Noble Creek to Noble Lake. Noble Creek is the stream by the south campground area. Follow the stream up the mountain until you meet the Pacific Crest Trail. Go left on the trail and zigzag up through the granite and sage. When you reach the top, Noble Lake is off to the right. What a beautiful spot! To my companions' horror, I actually jumped in and took a dip in the gelid water.

A less rigorous way to reach Noble Lake (although still a day hike) is to drive up to the top of Ebbetts Pass. Park at the summit or a couple hundred yards down the pass toward Silver Creek Campground, where there is a turnoff. The Pacific Crest Trail is marked. Head out under the pines. When I was last there, there was a bumper crop of lupine. Hike up through the mule ear, then down toward Noble Canyon and Noble Creek, through the hemlocks and pines to where the Noble Creek Trail from the campground hits the Pacific Crest Trail. From there, you just climb up to the top of Noble Canyon and see Noble Lake on the right.

A shorter hike is into Upper Kinney Lake. This is about 4 miles round-trip and takes off a couple hundred yards east of Ebbetts Pass. Find the Pacific Crest Trail sign on the north side of the road, which is where you'll start hiking. You'll see Lower Kinney Lake on the right, then find a split in the trail signed for Upper Kinney Lake. Go left. Find Upper Kinney Lake. This is a great place to spend the day. The hiking is easy (round-trip should take about two hours), and I saw an angler actually pull a nice-sized trout from the lake.

KEY INFORMATION

ADDRESS:	Silver Creek Campground Humboldt-Toiyabe National Forest Forest Supervisor 1200 Franklin Way Sparks, NV 89431
OPERATED BY:	U.S. Forest Service
INFORMATION:	(775) 331-6444; www.recreation.gov
OPEN:	Mid-June–mid-September (weather permitting)
SITES:	22 sites for tents and RVs
EACH SITE HAS:	Picnic table, fire ring
ASSIGNMENT:	Some sites are reservable, others are first come, first served
REGISTRATION:	At entrance; reserve by phone, (877) 444-6777, or online, www.reserveusa.com
FACILITIES:	Water, vault toilets, food locker
PARKING:	At individual site
FEE:	$13; $9 nonrefundable reservation fee
ELEVATION:	7,100 feet
RESTRICTIONS:	*Pets:* On leash only *Fires:* In fire ring *Alcohol:* No restrictions *Vehicles:* RVs up to 35 feet *Other:* Don't leave food out

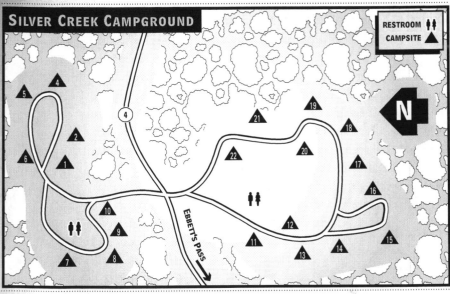

MAP

SILVER CREEK CAMPGROUND

RESTROOM
CAMPSITE

GETTING THERE

From Jackson, drive 52 miles east on CA 88 to the campground entrance on the right, past the Silver Lake dam.

GETTING THERE

From Markleeville, go 16 miles west on CA 4 to the campground. From Arnold, drive 46 miles east on CA 4 (over Ebbetts Pass) to the campground.

drift and buried himself up to his
the men were able to grab the
by his ears and drag him to safety.
ld off their trip until July, when more
nelted. Be sure to phone ahead, so
nd find the place snowed in.
, mention that you are tent-camping,
tent-only sites. These all seemed to
ighway than the RV-capacity sites.
n buying much more than ice and
everything else in from Jackson,

Many folks who stay at Silver Creek Campground are there for the fishing on Silver Creek and down on the Carson. Markleeville is convenient for supplies, and it also has a cute little museum. There's Grover Hot Springs State Park just west of Markleeville, with a swimming pool and hot springs, which are open for a small fee. You can also go the other way west of Ebbetts Pass and visit Upper and Lower Highland Lakes, or head farther west to Lake Alpine. (Upper and Lower Highland lakes and Lake Alpine appear in the entry for Upper and Lower Highland Lakes Campground.)

GPS COORDINATES

UTM Zone (WGS84) 10S

Easting 0750473

Northing 4284060

Latitude N 38° 40' 10.9849"

Longtitude W 120° 7' 15.6972"

GPS COORDINATES

UTM Zone (WGS84) 11S

Easting 0257340

Northing 4274770

Latitude N 38° 35' 17.7898"

Longtitude W 119° 47' 9.6863"

38
SILVER LAKE EAST CAMPGROUND

Silver Lake, Eldorado National Forest, near Kit Carson

SILVER LAKE IS A GREAT PLACE to bring a family. With resorts and another big campground nearby, there are always enough kids running around to entertain your own. The lake is a short walk away, where the kids congregate on the shore, and back at the campground the big boulders under the red firs draw youths like bees to honey. While the kids are off playing their own games, you can sit around and take it easy. It's prime camping!

And this area is beautiful. "Nothing in nature I am sure can present scenery more wild, more rugged, more bold, more romantic, and picturesquely beautiful than this mountain scenery." That's how one early pioneer described it. Now CA 88 is the Carson Pass Road, and it was Kit Carson who led Captain John Fremont, with his bodyguard of Delaware Native Americans, to the crest in 1844.

But it was the Mormon Brigade who engineered the wagon road. In fact, three of their numbers died in a Native American attack at Tragedy Springs, just southwest of Silver Lake. They were found naked in a shallow grave. The Native Americans probably killed them for their clothes. It is thought that many were inordinately fascinated with European clothing at the time—so fascinated, in fact, that it is rumored they would sometimes dig up the corpses of expired forty-niners to get their clothes, and would often contract whatever disease it was that had killed the unfortunate pilgrim in the first place.

If you come over the mountaintop from the west and look down at beautiful Silver Lake and the granite cliffs around it, you'll see that Silver Lake, like Caples Lake above it, is in a basin called a cirque. Cirques are formed when glaciers eat into the rock at its upper end. The ice slides down and takes the quarried rock with it, making room for more ice. Soon enough it digs out

> *A good place to bring kids, who will entertain each other while you relax.*

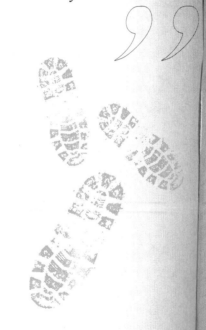

RATINGS

Beauty: ☆ ☆ ☆ ☆ ☆
Privacy: ☆ ☆ ☆
Spaciousness: ☆ ☆ ☆
Quiet: ☆ ☆ ☆
Security: ☆ ☆ ☆
Cleanliness: ☆ ☆ ☆ ☆

KEY INFORMATION

ADDRESS: Silver Lake East Campground Eldorado National Forest Forest Supervisor Amador Ranger District 26820 Silver Drive Pioneer, CA 95666

OPERATED BY: U.S. Forest Service

INFORMATION: (530) 622-5061, (209) 295-4251; www.fs.fed.us/r5/eldorado

OPEN: June–October 15 (depending on road and weather conditions)

SITES: 62 total; 35 tent; 27 tent, trailer, or RV

EACH SITE HAS: Picnic table, fireplace

ASSIGNMENT: 42 sites are reservable, 20 are first come, first served

REGISTRATION: At entrance; reserve by phone, (877) 444-6777, or online, www.recreation.gov

FACILITIES: Vault toilets, boat rental, potable water, campground store

PARKING: At individual site

FEE: $20–$22

ELEVATION: 7,200 feet

RESTRICTIONS: *Pets:* On leash only *Fires:* In fireplace *Alcohol:* No restrictions *Vehicles:* No bicycles on trails; sites limited to a maximum of 2 vehicles and 6 people *Other:* Don't leave food out; 14-day stay limit

a basin. Usually, these series called paternos Lake—so named beca beads in a rosary.

Fishing Silver L as heavily fished as voir or Caples Lake fine, since the lake are also boats for r brown, and rainbo headed for the no boat ramp, or the the American Ri bait shop for wh and where, and

While dad' ing. A great hik 3 miles round-t porating lunch 1.2 miles west the lodge if yo There's a sign up through th top of the rid wind are jun down throug the rock clif in the sun. non–polar

Anoth Granite L side of the Girls Car through shoes ar ous. Cro intersec Granite trail is Granit

P area i the M

MAP

SILVER L

RESTROOM
WATER ACCESS
HOST SITE

ELDORADO
FORE

donkey fell into ears. Fortunately afflicted donkey The Mormons he of the snow had r you don't arrive a

If you reserve because there are be farther off the Also, don't count beer locally—bring down the hill.

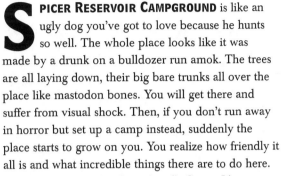

> *Ugly but fun—Spicer Reservoir Campground is a great place for canoeing, hiking, and exploring.*

SPICER **R**ESERVOIR **C**AMPGROUND is like an ugly dog you've got to love because he hunts so well. The whole place looks like it was made by a drunk on a bulldozer run amok. The trees are all laying down, their big bare trunks all over the place like mastodon bones. You will get there and suffer from visual shock. Then, if you don't run away in horror but set up a camp instead, suddenly the place starts to grow on you. You realize how friendly it all is and what incredible things there are to do here.

Come in off CA 4 from Angel's Camp. It's not a bad trip from Los Angeles, and it's easy to access from San Francisco and Sacramento. Stop in Angel's Camp if you have time—eat at the Gold Country Kitchen on Main, which sets out a good breakfast and lunch. Not far from here, a local, Bennager Rasberry, found gold when he was cleaning his muzzle-loader and accidentally discharged it into a manzanita bush. The blast revealed gold hanging on the bush roots. The boom was on.

Continue on CA 4 toward Spicer, up past Arnold (the last good supply point for groceries, fast food, and supplies), to unfortunate Tamarack, where FS 7N01 (signed Spicer Reservoir Road) takes off to the south. Poor little Tamarack holds the world record for snowfall in one winter—73.5 feet. Imagine. That's 25 yards of snow—12 men standing one on top of another. That's why God invented skis and snowshoes and why rabbits have such big feet.

It's about 8 miles to the campground. You'll pass Stanislaus River Campground about 4 miles in on the right. Check it out. The sites are along the river, among the trees. If the river is not up at spring flood, this is a great place to camp. Kids love it. It is great wading (bring water booties), and there are pools where the water backs up, warms up, and makes a wonderful place to dip in on a hot summer's day.

RATINGS

Beauty: ☆
Privacy: ☆ ☆ ☆
Spaciousness: ☆ ☆ ☆
Quiet: ☆ ☆ ☆
Security: ☆ ☆ ☆ ☆
Cleanliness: ☆ ☆ ☆ ☆

Drive another 4 miles to Spicer Reservoir Campground. Take a look at the water. A huge part of it—the long finger in the canyon to the east—is for nonmotorized boats only. This makes it perfect for canoes or kayaks (even small sailboats). It gets a little breezy up there to use the small inflatables, unless you don't mind being stranded over on one side or another of the reservoir. Rent canoes or kayaks for the weekend in the flatland and cartop them up to Spicer. Once you paddle the canyon that pushes its way into the Carson Iceberg Wilderness, you'll want to own your own craft. Many rental places let you take the weekend rental off the purchase price of something new.

Right from the campground you can hike the 10 miles down to Sand Flat. Only a walking fool could turn around and go back up in one day, so arrange a car shuttle (although it's a long way around via Sonora or the passes), or take a sleeping bag down with you and spend the night at Sand Flat Campground. There are good sites down by the stream. It's best to hike halfway to Corral Meadow and come back to camp. The trail is not too difficult, and the scenery is incredible—an ocean of granite with bursts of wildflowers in the meadows.

Another great hike is up to Rock Lake. Drive back to FS 7N01. Head right, 4 miles, to the trailhead marked Elephant Rock Lake. The trail splits immediately. Go right. The second time the trail splits, you can go left to see Elephant Rock Lake—pretty, with lily pads and flowers on the shore. Go right around the shore to get back on the Rock Lake Trail. Go straight through pines and fir and hit another split in the trail. Go straight and climb up into Carson Iceberg Wilderness and the Sea of Granite. You should reach Rock Lake in an easy hour's hike (about 2 miles).

I never get beyond Rock Lake. This is such a great place to have lunch and swim. There are little rock islands all over the place on which you can beach yourself and loll in the sun like a walrus. Bring a pair of water booties, as the lake is shallow and it's fun to splash around.

Or, I was told, you can also make a loop back to the trailhead, which is a longer hike by a mile or two. Go past Rock Lake to a junction for Highland Lakes.

ADDRESS:	Spicer Reservoir Campground Stanislaus National Forest Calaveras Ranger District P.O. Box 500 Hathaway Pines, CA 95233
OPERATED BY:	U.S. Forest Service
INFORMATION:	(209) 795-1381; www.fs.fed.us/r5/stanislaus
OPEN:	June–October (depending on road and weather conditions)
SITES:	60 sites for tents or RVs
EACH SITE HAS:	Picnic table, fireplace, grill
ASSIGNMENT:	First come, first served; no reservations
REGISTRATION:	At entrance
FACILITIES:	Water, vault toilets
PARKING:	At individual site
FEE:	$20
ELEVATION:	6,200 feet
RESTRICTIONS:	*Pets:* On leash only *Fires:* In fireplace *Alcohol:* No restrictions *Vehicles:* RVs and trailers allowed up to 50 feet *Other:* Don't leave food out; 14-day stay limit

MAP

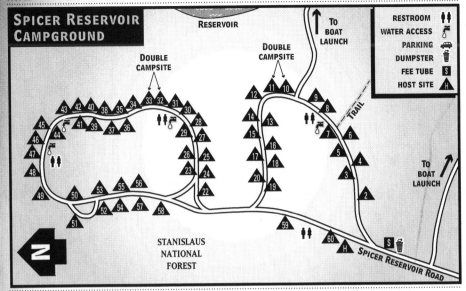

SPICER RESERVOIR CAMPGROUND

RESERVOIR

To BOAT LAUNCH

DOUBLE CAMPSITE

DOUBLE CAMPSITE

TRAIL

RESTROM		
WATER ACCESS		
PARKING		
DUMPSTER		
FEE TUBE	S	
HOST SITE	H	

To BOAT LAUNCH

STANISLAUS NATIONAL FOREST

SPICER RESERVOIR ROAD

N

GETTING THERE

From Angel's Camp, go 32 miles east on Ebbetts Pass Road (CA 4) to Spicer Reservoir Road (FS 7N01), and turn right. The campground is 8 miles south.

Go right here to another junction, where you go right for Summit Lake. Follow the signs for Summit Lake until you cross FS 7N01, which you took in to the trailhead. Go right and walk up the road to your car.

I found Spicer Reservoir Campground to be a good base for further adventuring. In addition to canoeing and hiking the trail, I liked hiking around the reservoir. There's an angler's trail part of the way, and then you have to scramble, but the granite makes for good traction on your hands and seat of your pants. Spicer also makes a good first camp for dispersed camping up along the roads to Utica and Union reservoirs. You can get drinking water and use the telephone down at Spicer.

GPS COORDINATES

UTM Zone (WGS84) 10S

Easting 0757811

Northing 4256786

Latitude N 38° 25' 19.7362"

Longtitude W 120° 2' 48.6852"

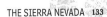

THIS CAMPGROUND IS MY FAVORITE campground in the Sierra Nevada. At 8,600 feet, the campsites are by the pretty Highland Lakes, in a valley full of bright wildflowers. If you can get in on the road to Highland Lakes, it means the snowdrifts have melted. If the snowdrifts have melted, you know the wildflowers are out—this is a short season. To the north, even in late August, Folger Peak has snow fields. Hiram Peak to the south is as big and brown as a warm bear. There are hikes going everywhere. This is off the beaten track. You don't just happen to show up there, so plan to stay for a while.

The Highland Lakes are up on the west side of Ebbetts Pass. This area is notorious for snow. Some years the pass is snowed in until August. In July 1995 the snow at Lake Alpine, a thousand feet farther down, drifted 30 feet deep. Pacific storms get sucked in through the Golden Gate and head east to the Sierra Nevada below Ebbetts Pass. At about 7,000 feet, the clouds cool down and dump all their moisture as snow. Lots of snow.

Well, it's not much easier going now until the drifts melt, and the county plows the road, and the days get warm, and flowers bloom in the meadows, and planted fish run in the streams. The dirt road in off CA 4 is rough-going but easily managed by even the wimpiest of sedans. Just go slowly and mind the bumps. It takes off to the southeast just 1 mile below Ebbetts Pass (14.5 miles above Lake Alpine). The road (FS 8N01) goes down a steep hill, then runs along pretty Highland Creek filled with wonderful places for dispersed camping, if you thought ahead for the requisite permit (free at any ranger station) and have a bucket and shovel for fire suppression. Some of the area is designated Rehabilitation Project, meaning you can walk in and enjoy, carry in a tent and camp, but

> *Come prepared to stay—this is my favorite Sierra Nevada campground.*

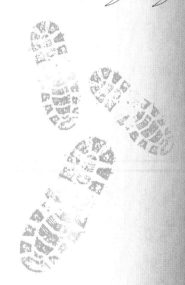

RATINGS

Beauty: ✿ ✿ ✿ ✿ ✿
Privacy: ✿ ✿ ✿ ✿ ✿
Spaciousness: ✿ ✿ ✿ ✿ ✿ ✿
Quiet: ✿ ✿ ✿ ✿ ✿
Security: ✿ ✿ ✿ ✿ ✿
Cleanliness: ✿ ✿ ✿ ✿ ✿

ADDRESS:	Upper and Lower Highland Lakes Campground Stanislaus National Forest Forest Supervisor 19777 Greenley Road Sonora, CA 95370
OPERATED BY:	U.S. Forest Service
INFORMATION:	(209) 532-3671; www.fs.fed.us/r5/stanislaus
OPEN:	Late June–October (weather permitting)
SITES:	35 sites for tents
EACH SITE HAS:	Picnic table, fireplace
ASSIGNMENT:	First come, first served; no reservations
REGISTRATION:	At entrance
FACILITIES:	Hand-pump well water, vault toilets
PARKING:	At individual site
FEE:	$8
ELEVATION:	8,600 feet
RESTRICTIONS:	*Pets:* On leash only *Fires:* In fireplace *Alcohol:* No restrictions *Vehicles:* Large RVs or trailers not recommended *Other:* Don't leave food out; 14-day stay limit

you can't drive your vehicle in. Of course, where it is not posted you can drive in on existing access roads and camp by your car.

Pass fields of purple lupine and crazy shooting stars and a wonderful old-style line ranch, and after a steep climb there are the two Highland Lakes and the Lower Highland Lake Campground on the right, under lightning-blasted pines. The sites are not well designed, but they are pretty and clean. There's one outhouse near the middle of camp, and a pump for water across from site 10. Remember to bring a bucket for hauling water from the pump to your campsite.

To reach the Upper Highland Lakes part of the campground, take the dirt road that goes west between the two lakes. It has a confusing sign that appears to advise four-wheel-drive only. Ignore this. The road to the camp area (only a few hundred yards long) is just like the road you drove in on. Any sedan can make it easily. These sites are just above the lakes in a stand of pines. Right away, you'll see the pump and outhouse. The campsites are back in under the pines and a short walk from the Upper Highland Lake. If you want privacy, camp up here. If you have kids who want to run around, or if you like the western sun to warm your bones, camp in the Lower Highland Lakes area below, where it is sunnier and flatter.

Bring supplies. The nearest store is at Lake Alpine, or east to Markleeville. Bring an extra cooler filled with ice, and duct-tape the top. Leave coolers in the shade. Put a wet cloth over the coolers and let evaporation cool the outsides. Think about buying one of those coolers you can fold up afterward as an extra. Bring water booties for the lake. Think about bringing a little inflatable Sevylor-style boat (at chain stores everywhere for $50 or less) to float around in with a book and fishing gear (brook trout). Buy a Lake Alpine Carson–Iceberg Wilderness map for $1.95 at the Lake Alpine store so you can navigate the trails around the lakes. (Or buy the more ambitious Forest Service map at any nearby ranger station.) Remember sunscreen, as the air is thin and the sun strong. Remember to bring lip balm and skin lotion, as it is dry. Bring cotton balls if the kids tend to have nose bleeds (good for staunch-

MAP

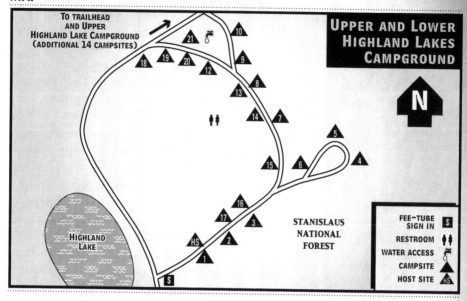

ing the flow). Borrow from the other campers if you forget anything—most campers are friendly and are willing to help by lending things that they prudently remembered to bring along.

Camping at Upper and Lower Highland Lakes Campground requires a little extra forethought and travel time. But it's worth it. Remember, phone ahead to get road conditions, to find out whether the campground is open, and to see if drinking water is available. If there is no drinking water, boil lake water (five minutes at a roiling boil), or buy a water filter from a camping store.

GETTING THERE

From Arnold, go 29 miles east on CA 4 to Lake Alpine. Continue 15 miles past the Lake Alpine store to FS 8N01 (signed to Highland Lakes) on the right. At this point, you will be 1 mile west of Ebbetts Pass. Drive 7.5 miles in on a graded dirt road.

GPS COORDINATES

UTM Zone (WGS84) 11S

Easting 0255188

Northing 4263755

Latitude N 38° 29' 18.7150"

Longtitude W 119° 48' 24.6384"

> An experience in style and gentility— only the bears are rowdy.

DRIVE INTO **M**OHAWK **V**ALLEY on your way to Upper Jamison Campground, and all of a sudden you are in the land of lush green golf courses and condos. Graeagle, just 5 miles from the park, is a retirement mecca, with elegant restaurants, a good grocery store, a deli with smoked meats, and a pond with a great swimming beach right in the center of town.

The nearby Feather River Inn used to be the most fashionable resort in northern California. Passengers arrived on the train, and porters pushed their steamer trunks over in wheelbarrows. Now the flannels and black cocktail dresses with pearls have given way to ski parkas or golf shirts, depending on the season, but the area still has a sense of style and gentility.

Drive into Plumas-Eureka State Park. The rangers are polite and friendly. Everything is tasteful and under control. The museum is thoughtfully done. The handout pamphlets are grammatically correct. Drive another mile or so to the Upper Jamison Campground at the end of the road. By pretty Little Jamison Creek, the campsites are well separated and nicely screened from one another by trees. The bathrooms are rough but clean. The whole camping experience is enjoyable, though a little removed. Maybe it's the area's rich history that gives you the Westminster Abbey feeling of strolling among the bones of kings and commoners whose hopes, dreams, and sins are now all dust.

Indeed, except for nearby Jamison City's (now Johnsville) brief raffish period replete with fisticuffs and fancy women, the area has always been respectable. Johnsville was a company mining town with solid citizens brought in from Wales, Austria, and elsewhere, to work the mines and live in harmony in the company town (now all buried in the local Johnsville cemetery—worth a visit).

RATINGS

Beauty: ✩ ✩ ✩ ✩
Privacy: ✩ ✩ ✩ ✩
Spaciousness: ✩ ✩ ✩ ✩
Quiet: ✩ ✩ ✩
Security: ✩ ✩ ✩ ✩ ✩
Cleanliness: ✩ ✩ ✩ ✩

Only the bears are rude. Folks are implored to cooperate with the rangers to keep those naughty ursines in line. Don't leave food around while you are not in the area. Keep a clean camp. Put your food and coolers in your trunk when you do leave. If you have a hatchback, disguise the coolers with a blanket or haphazardly placed clothes. Bears are smart, strong, and very hungry. They have been known to tear open an automobile like a sardine can, just to get a tube of sunscreen.

Naturally, we were there for two days and didn't see a bear. We did see the work of beavers up at Madora Lake, as well as Canada geese, coots, and a glimpse of what might have been a fox around dusk on our walk. Directions to Madora Lake are quite clear in the Plumas-Eureka State Park handout. In fact, you passed the turnoff to the lake on your way in from Graeagle.

Walking in and around Madora Lake takes about an hour. On the far side of the lake is a picnic table, perfect for a sandwich or a sundowner while you look for beaver. This industrious rodent practically fueled the western exploration. During the late 1700s and early 1800s, explorers headed west as they decimated the eastern beaver population. They cured the pelts and sent them to factories where the hair was made into felt, which was then made into beaver top hats. These hats held their shape and repelled water, and were all the rage for a while.

Now the beavers have aggressively bounced back and can be seen around Plumas-Eureka State Park (another sure beaver sighting hotspot is Lake Earl Wildlife Area just north of Crescent City). Beavers like streams around aspen, birch, alder, and willows. They come out most in the summer after the birth of their kits, and work mainly in the early morning and evening.

Another great hike is up the Grass Lake Trail, where you will find even more beaver signs. Grass Lake is pretty and surrounded by Jeffrey pine and red fir. Work your way around to the west side of the lake to get the best view of the incredible mountains on the other side.

KEY INFORMATION

ADDRESS: Upper Jamison Campground Plumas-Eureka State Park 310 Johnsville Road Blairsden, CA 96103

OPERATED BY: California State Parks

INFORMATION: (530) 836-2380; www.parks.ca.gov

OPEN: May–October (until it snows)

SITES: 67 sites for tents, trailers, or RVs; 14 walk-in sites

EACH SITE HAS: Picnic table, fireplace, bear-proof lockers

ASSIGNMENT: Reservations Memorial Day–Labor Day; www.reserveamerica.com or (800) 444-PARK (7275); rest of the year is first come, first served

REGISTRATION: At office in museum by entrance

FACILITIES: Water, flush toilets, hot showers, wood for sale

PARKING: At individual site

FEE: $20

ELEVATION: 5,200 feet

RESTRICTIONS: *Pets:* On leash only
Fires: In fireplace
Alcohol: No restrictions
Vehicles: RVs and trailers up to 30 feet
Other: No burning of dead or downed wood—purchased firewood only

MAP

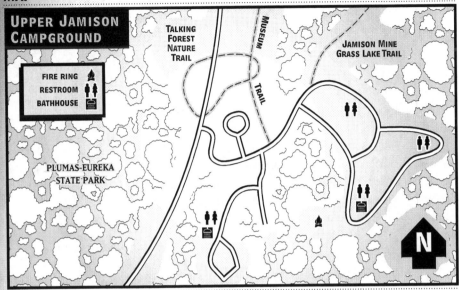

GETTING THERE

From Graeagle, take CA 89 north to CA 70. Take CA 70 west to County Road A14. Five miles west on CR A14 is Plumas-Eureka State Park. Go left past Park Headquarters to the campground at the end of the road.

Don't miss camping at Plumas-Eureka. But remember, Upper Jamison Campground is first come, first served, so plan accordingly. Pay your fee in the office in the museum if you arrive before closing time; otherwise, just drive down to the campground, occupy a site, and pay the fee the next morning when the charming ranger comes around in her truck.

GPS COORDINATES

UTM Zone (WGS84) 10S
Easting 0696464
Northing 4401465
Latitude N 39° 44' 25.6454"
Longtitude W 120° 42' 25.8086"

WA KA LUU HEP YOO CAMPGROUND

WA KA LUU HEP YOO (sometimes spelled Wakaluu Hepyoo) means "wild river" in the Native American dialect Miwuk. The campground sits on a sloping bank above the Stanislaus River, in woods where the Miwuk people lived seasonally for more than 2,000 years. Wa Ka Luu Hep Yoo hosts incredibly nice camping, yet still preserves historic Miwuk features, including grinding stones and middens. It's a great cultural experience, accentuated by campground signs in both English and Miwuk.

Wa Ka Luu Hep Yoo would be a wonderful campground even without its location on the Stanislaus River, but the large rushing waterway boosts the camping experience to the upper echelon of California tent pitching. Downslope from the campsites, the river is easily reached by a paved and dirt-trail network that threads through the campground. Fishing is popular, and although signs warn about strong currents and drownings, on a hot day it's nearly impossible to resist taking a dip in the pristine, crystal-clear, cool water. Use good sense here: if you want to take the plunge, stick to the deep, placid pools and away from the shallows where the current is strongest, and keep small children out of the river. Giant rock slabs lining the river make perfect lounges for basking in the sun. It's a 5-mile, class-IV whitewater trip from the raft access at the Sourgrass day-use lot (across the river from the campground) to Calaveras Big Trees State Park (phone the ranger station for current conditions and permit information).

The campground's 49 sites are situated along a balloon-shaped access road. A handful of RV sites sit near the showers at the front of the campground, and the remaining sites are oriented to tents. About half the sites require a walk, ranging from a few steps to a few hundred yards. The remaining sites are the traditional

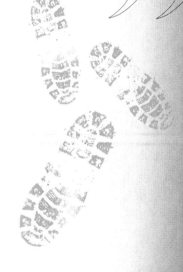

> *Constructed in 1999, this well-planned campground is nestled in woods above the Stanislaus River.*

RATINGS

Beauty: ✰ ✰ ✰ ✰ ✰
Privacy: ✰ ✰ ✰ ✰
Spaciousness: ✰ ✰ ✰ ✰
Quiet: ✰ ✰ ✰ ✰ ✰
Security: ✰ ✰ ✰ ✰ ✰
Cleanliness: ✰ ✰ ✰ ✰ ✰

ADDRESS: Wa Ka Luu Hep Yoo
Campground
Calaveras Ranger
District, Stanislaus
National Forest,
P.O. Box 500,
Hathaway Pines, CA
95233

OPERATED BY: Stanislaus National
Forest

INFORMATION: (209) 795-1381;
www.fs.fed.us/5r/
stanislaus

OPEN: June–October,
weather permitting

SITES: 49; 27 are walk-in
sites

EACH SITES HAS: Picnic table,
fire ring

ASSIGNMENT: First come, first
served; no
reservations

REGISTRATION: Self-register at
information area
near showers,
at front of camp-
ground

FACILITIES: Flush and vault
toilets, hot showers,
drinking water

PARKING: At individual sites,
and in small lots
for walk-in sites

FEE: $16

ELEVATION: 3,900 feet

RESTRICTIONS: *Pets:* Dogs must be
leashed
Fires: In established
pits/rings only
Alcohol: No
restrictions
Vehicles: Maximum
vehicle length
50 feet
Other: 14-day
stay limit

park-and-unpack style, with a few adjacent sites perfect for two families or small groups (the campground limit is six people to a site). All sites have fire pits with grills and big picnic tables. The vegetation in the campground is primarily ponderosa pines, black and live oaks, and cedars. There is little understory vegetation to screen views of the campsites, although some sites are shielded by massive boulders.

With a little effort, you can camp at what we consider the nicest sites, 15 and 16. These require the longest walks but are the closest to the river—perfect if you've come to fish for rainbow and brown trout. The walk-in sites nearest the river offer little privacy but are well-spaced. When we camped at Wa Ka Luu Hep Yoo on a Sunday night in early June, only one of the walk-in sites was occupied. The camp host recommended sites 41 and 42, quiet, shaded sites at the back of the campground loop, but we chose site 33, which required a short walk but provided a big payoff—partial views down to the river and a mixture of shade and sunshine. Since we were partly out of the woods, there was great star-gazing on a clear, comfortable night. And in the morning, after three nights of camping, the hot showers (free for campers) were most appreciated!

A very rough fire road departs from the Sourgrass day-use lot on a 2-mile journey to Pine Needle Flat—from our campsite we watched a few four-wheel-drive vehicles struggling back to Boards Crossing Road. Note that the trail is open to hiking, mountain biking, and limited off-highway-vehicle use. For a more sedate hiking experience, make the short drive to the sequoia groves at Calaveras Big Trees State Park (see listing). If you want to stretch your legs but not really hike, take an easy stroll through the campground and under the bridge, to a lookout above a roaring section of the Stanislaus. The Calaveras Ranger District hosts interpretive programs in the summer months, including basket weaving, Miwuk plant use, and Miwuk songs. Look for grinding stones, bowl-shaped depressions in boulders where Miwuks worked acorns into meal, in the campground—there's one in a fenced area near site 7. The camp host is friendly and knowledgeable about the campground and the surrounding area, if you have

MAP

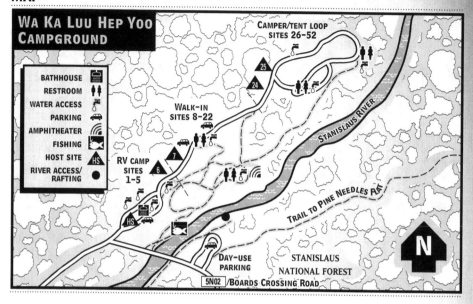

WA KA LUU HEP YOO CAMPGROUND

CAMPER/TENT LOOP
SITES 26–52

BATHHOUSE
RESTROOM
WATER ACCESS
PARKING
AMPHITHEATER
FISHING
HOST SITE
RIVER ACCESS/
RAFTING

WALK-IN
SITES 8–22

RV CAMP
SITES
1–5

STANISLAUS RIVER

TRAIL TO PINE NEEDLES RD

DAY-USE
PARKING

STANISLAUS
NATIONAL FOREST

5N02 / BOARDS CROSSING ROAD

N

questions—he's been at Wa Ka Luu Hep Yoo since the campground opened in 1999.

Wa Ka Luu Hep Yoo is set in a relatively low elevation, unlike the popular campgrounds 20 miles or so farther up CA 4, including the Lake Alpine area, where elevations range from 6,000 to 8,000 feet. Since the temperature drops about three degrees for every 1,000 feet gained, Wa Ka Luu Hep Yoo is slightly warmer than the campgrounds at Spicer Reservoir and Pine Marten (see listings). If you're averse to heat, check out Wa Ka Luu Hep Yoo in autumn.

Arnold and Murphys are the two largest towns on the way to the campground, with grocery and hardware stores, restaurants, gas, and sporting-goods shops (remember you'll need a fishing license if you plan to try your luck for trout). Dorrington and Camp Connell have limited services, but you can pick up ice and other camping staples at their general stores. Wine production is on the steady increase in this part of the state, and high-quality vintages from nearby wineries are available, even from the general stores in the area.

GETTING THERE

From Angel's Camp on CA 49 in Calaveras County, turn east onto CA 4. Drive east 25 miles to the small settlement of Dorrington, then turn right onto Boards Crossing Road. Follow Boards Crossing Road south 5 miles, then turn left into the campground.

GPS COORDINATES

UTM Zone (WGS84) 10S

Easting 0741595

Northing 4243282

Latitude N 38° 18' 18.4427"

Longtitude W 120° 14' 13.2974"

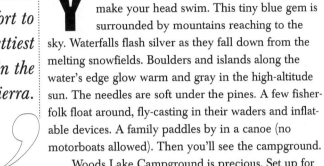

> *Make an effort to camp here—the prettiest lake camping in the High Sierra.*

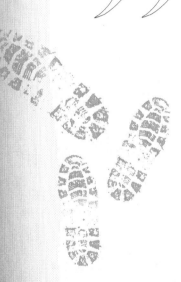

YOUR FIRST LOOK AT **WOODS LAKE** will make your head swim. This tiny blue gem is surrounded by mountains reaching to the sky. Waterfalls flash silver as they fall down from the melting snowfields. Boulders and islands along the water's edge glow warm and gray in the high-altitude sun. The needles are soft under the pines. A few fisherfolk float around, fly-casting in their waders and inflatable devices. A family paddles by in a canoe (no motorboats allowed). Then you'll see the campground.

Woods Lake Campground is precious. Set up for tent campers, the first 14 or so sites have the fireplace and picnic table set well back from the parking space. You'll pitch your tent among the red penstamen–emblazoned rocks, or down in a hollow, or up on a hillside. You have to come Sunday afternoon through Thursday to get a spot here. People come back year after year. One woman has been coming with her daughter for 20 years. Eagerly, she asked me which site I'd found. When I told her, she said, "Oh, that's where we brought her [indicating her lovely college-aged daughter] when she was first born."

Think about water. Woods Lake Campground is plumbed for water, but there has been a failure of some kind. So the only available water is a 180-foot-deep well accessed by a hand pump in front of campsite 18. It takes two to pump water. One vigorously manipulates the handle (it takes about 20 pumps to bring up the water), while the other person holds the water jug. It's not a bad idea to bring a bucket or a funnel, since the water comes out of the pump spigot in a way that makes it difficult to direct it into a narrow-neck jug. You work for it, but the water is so sweet.

I arrived with my older sister from the East Coast, and we immediately trekked around the lake in our go-aheads (flip-flops). Good thing, too, since where the

RATINGS

Beauty: ✪ ✪ ✪ ✪ ✪
Privacy: ✪ ✪ ✪ ✪ ✪
Spaciousness: ✪ ✪ ✪ ✪ ✪
Quiet: ✪ ✪ ✪ ✪
Security: ✪ ✪ ✪ ✪ ✪
Cleanliness: ✪ ✪ ✪ ✪ ✪

waterfalls ran into the lake you had to wade knee-deep to cross. Then there was the swamp on the far side of the lake, which we avoided by climbing up over the rocks and down the other side, risking life and limb to cross yet another quickly moving stream before we found the trail back to the campground.

There are two trailheads near the campground. From either, you make a big arc through Winnemucca Lake, Round Top Lake, and back down to Woods Lake. The full trip is about 5 miles. Remember to watch the weather—it can snow here just about any time. It's not a bad thing to carry one of those emergency rain parkas (buy them in a camping store) in your pack, along with your sweater, which could give you a margin of comfort if it does start storming.

Access one end of the trail from the day-use parking lot near Woods Lake. Cross the bridge over the stream and follow the signed trail to Winnemucca Lake. At first you'll walk on the shoulder of a moraine (a ridge of rubble left by a retreating glacier), then into a pine forest. Spot the arrasta (a Mexican mining device for breaking up ore) on the right. Then the trail breaks out into an incredible meadow filled with acres of wildflowers tumbling up toward the ridge and sky above. What an incredible sight! Only later when we chatted with a nice woman hiking with a huge slobbering hound did we learn that this wildflower spot is famous for its display.

Soon enough you'll come to Winnemucca Lake (named for a Paiute chief from Nevada), a sharp blue shard of water set in weathered gray granite. Two daring young hikers hastily breast-stroked across to a warm boulder and flopped up on it like pink seals. Otherwise, there was just the sigh of the wind across the rocks and stunted pines.

A four-by-four signpost directs you to Round Top Lake. There's more huffing and puffing to this lake, then the trail swings down around Lost Cabin Mine (posted against trespassers) and drops you at the campground near sites 14 through 16.

Fishing at Woods Lake and Winnemucca Lake is fine. I saw a few folks down at Woods Lake pull in some ten-inch rainbows at the Woods Creek end of the

KEY INFORMATION

ADDRESS:	Woods Lake Campground Eldorado National Forest Amador Ranger District 26820 Silver Drive Pioneer, CA 95666
OPERATED BY:	U.S. Forest Service
INFORMATION:	(530) 644-6048, (209) 295-4251; www.fs.fed.us/r5/eldorado
OPEN:	June 15–October 15 (weather permitting)
SITES:	25 sites for tents; 8 wheelchair-accessible
EACH SITE HAS:	Picnic table, fireplace
ASSIGNMENT:	First come, first served; no reservations
REGISTRATION:	At entrance
FACILITIES:	Piped well water, vault toilets, boat rental, campground store, picnic area
PARKING:	At individual site
FEE:	$22; $5 extra vehicle
ELEVATION:	8,200 feet
RESTRICTIONS:	*Pets:* On leash only *Fires:* In fireplace *Alcohol:* No restrictions *Vehicles:* No RVs or trailers, 2 vehicles and 6 people maximum per site *Other:* Don't leave food out, use bear boxes; 14-day stay limit

MAP

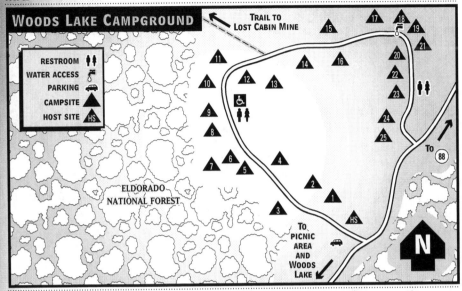

WOODS LAKE CAMPGROUND

TRAIL TO
LOST CABIN MINE

| RESTROOM |
| WATER ACCESS |
| PARKING |
| CAMPSITE |
| HOST SITE | HS |

ELDORADO
NATIONAL FOREST

To
88

To
PICNIC
AREA
AND
WOODS
LAKE

N

GETTING THERE

From Jackson, drive east
70 miles on CA 88, past
Caples Lake, to the turnoff to
Woods Lake Campground on
the right. Go about 2 miles.
The campground entrance
is on the right before you
reach Woods Lake.

lake. But fishing here is not about what you catch, obviously. It is a religious experience, and most people seemed to approach it that way.

The little Carson Pass Information Center a few miles east on CA 88 is worth visiting—at least to see what books and pamphlets they have about the area. Read too the plaque outside about old Snowshoe Thompson. This old boy was tough as nails and makes our iron men of today look like a bunch of wimps.

Remember to bring supplies. Caples Lake Resort has a tiny store that sells ice, beer, and fishing gear, but not much else. The nearest real grocery store is across the pass at Woodfords. For campers who strike out at Woods Lake, I suggest going over the pass to the Blue Lakes.

GPS COORDINATES

UTM Zone (WGS84) 10S
Easting 0759987
Northing 4286177
Latitude N 38° 41' 9.7115"
Longtitude W 120° 0' 39.6718"

44
WRIGHTS LAKE
CAMPGROUND

RESERVE YOUR SITE months ahead. Bring the kids, because Wrights Lake Campground is perfect for kids of all ages. The lake is clean and warm, ideal for swimming off the rocks and shore, or from canoes and small inflatables on the water. This is a made-to-order movie set for a coming-of-age film. The campground is small and intimate. For once the tent-only sites get the best real estate—down by the lake—while the RVers are off on the other side of the dam. The sites are private, with boulders and coppices of pines blocking them from one another. The plateau area that Wrights Lake occupies is sylvan and warm, with crisscrossing streams—more meadow than the harsher oceans of granite farther south toward Yosemite.

This place is popular—everybody has a smile on their face. Folks from Sacramento and San Francisco plan a year ahead to spend their vacations here. All you can hear is the sound of birds singing and the kids splashing into the water and laughing. Even the campground's namesake was a happy guy. Friends on an expedition in 1881 wrote about James William Albert Wright: "Captain Wright was the only fleshy member of our party. His ribs were so encased in such thick layers of fatty tissue that, knowing his inability to freeze, we elected that he should sleep on the windward side of the camp."

You have to bring some kind of flotation device along. Motorboats are not allowed, so midnight paddles are a widespread Wrights Lake practice. Light rooftop canoes or kayaks are best adapted to the lake, but any inflatable will do. Go for one of the Sevylor-style jobs for about $50 in Big 5 or Sportmart. Buy an electric pump to plug into your car's cigarette lighter, and a repair kit. These inflatables are fun on high mountain lakes. They get you out of the freezing water, off the shore, and into the sun.

> *Reserve ahead—this is the best place to bring kids. It is stunningly beautiful, too.*

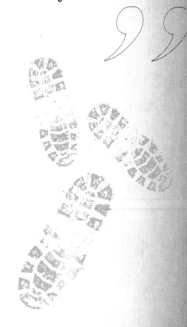

RATINGS

Beauty: ✪ ✪ ✪ ✪ ✪
Privacy: ✪ ✪ ✪
Spaciousness: ✪ ✪ ✪
Quiet: ✪ ✪ ✪
Security: ✪ ✪ ✪
Cleanliness: ✪ ✪ ✪

ADDRESS: Wrights Lake
Campground
Pacific Ranger
District
7887 Highway 50
Pollock Pines, CA
95726

OPERATED BY: U.S. Forest Service

INFORMATION: (530) 644-2349;
www.fs.fed.us/r5/
eldorado

OPEN: June–October
(depending on
road and weather
conditions)

SITES: 68 total; 44 tent,
24 tent or RV,
2 family sites

EACH SITE HAS: Picnic table, fireplace

ASSIGNMENT: First come, first
served; reservations
recommended

REGISTRATION: At entrance; reserve
by phone, (877) 444-
6777, or online,
www.recreation.gov

FACILITIES: Water, vault toilets

PARKING: At individual site

FEE: $20; $36 for double
site, $5 extra vehi-
cle, $9 nonrefund-
able reservation fee

ELEVATION: 7,000 feet

RESTRICTIONS: *Pets:* On leash only
Fires: In fireplace
Alcohol: No
restrictions
Vehicles: RVs up
to 22 feet; motor-
boats prohibited
Other: Don't leave
food out; 14-day
stay limit

Wrights Lake is accessed from US 50. Once called the Placerville Road, US 50 was built as a toll road by Colonel John Calhoun (Cock-Eye) Johnson. He made a ton of money on wagons heading for Virginia City (well worth a visit—go on a weekday). Cock-Eye's toll road was rumored to be "five-feet-deep by a hundred-and-thirty-miles long, and composed mostly of mountains, snow, and mud." Now cars and buses (gambler's specials) fly up and down this road. It's kind of unnerving, and you'll need to watch carefully for the Wrights Lake Road, which comes abruptly on a curve, so be mindful of the frantic traffic.

Bring lots of ice and supplies. The nearest reliable gasoline, ice, and grocery towns are in Meyers to the east over Echo Summit, or Riverton to the west. Bring an extra cooler packed with ice and duct-taped shut. Put a wet blanket on it and cool it by evaporation. Put drinks in a little six-pack cooler so folks won't be opening and closing the food cooler all day long. Make a menu and stick to it—it's amazing how little food you need if it is planned out. Don't count on "living off the lake," although people do catch rainbow and brown trout—it is stocked, and some of the brown trout that survive through the winter get to be pretty big boys.

Hiking around Wrights Lake is fun. Many of the other day hikes require permits, which you can conveniently get at the Wrights Lake Campground. The last time I was up there, we hiked up to Smith Lake. The hike is a killer but has the asset of leaving from the campground. Just hike up the road on the east side of Wrights Lake to the Twin and Grouse Lake Trailhead. Cross the fence and walk up through the meadow. At the beginning of July it was packed with flowers.

After maybe half a mile, the trail splits. Go right up the slope. The trail climbs. Pass a sign for the Desolation Wilderness, and go right when the trail splits. When you reach a trail signed for Twin/Island Lake, go right again. This climb is a bear, until you get to Grouse Lake. If you have any sand left in you, go left around the shore and follow the trail through the swamp, up to Hemlock Lake.

Keep going to the right of Hemlock Lake and stagger on up the mountain to Smith Lake. This lake is

MAP

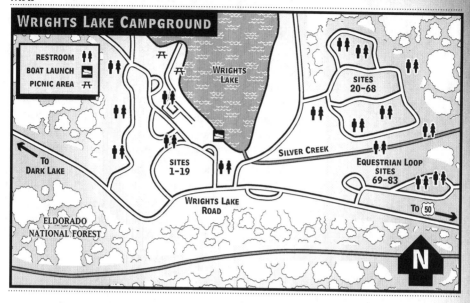

WRIGHTS LAKE CAMPGROUND

RESTROOM
BOAT LAUNCH
PICNIC AREA

WRIGHTS LAKE

SITES 20-68

To DARK LAKE

SILVER CREEK

SITES 1-19

EQUESTRIAN LOOP SITES 69-83

WRIGHTS LAKE ROAD

To 50

ELDORADO NATIONAL FOREST

N

good dipping, and you're going to need it. You've only walked 4 miles from the campground, but 3 of them have been straight up. Imagine how you'd feel if you were carrying a 50-pound pack. No wonder John Muir went hiking in his great coat with all his provisions in his pockets.

GETTING THERE

From Placerville, drive 34 miles east on US 50. Turn left on Wrights Lake Road (watch the turn—it's dangerous), and go 8 miles up the narrow road to the campground.

GPS COORDINATES

UTM Zone (WGS84) 10S

Easting 0740054

Northing 4303147

Latitude N 38° 50' 39.8977"

Longtitude W 120° 14' 2.5188"

> *Bring your fishing pole, bathing suit, and anything that floats.*

FIRST OFF, NOTE THAT Little Grass Valley Reservoir is not in the outskirts of the gold country town of Grass Valley. It's not even in the same county. Little Grass Valley Reservoir, a 1,615-acre man-made lake nestled in the mountains of Plumas County, collects water from the Feather River watershed. Wyandotte is one of six campgrounds around the reservoir. Sites at Red Feather, Running Deer, and Horse Camp are reservable, while Wyandotte, Peninsula Tent, and Black Rock are not. Peninsula Tent is a good option if Wyandotte is full; Peninsula Tent has forested walk-in sites a short distance from the lake but sits right off the lake access road and can be a bit noisy. Wyandotte is more scenic and peaceful.

The sites at Wyandotte are situated along a straight road, with two tiny loops at either end. The campground slopes uphill from the shoreline, with sites at the lower end (21 through 29) offering the closest lake access, via a short path, to one of the reservoir's boat ramps and the shoreline. Some of the sites in the upper part of the campground offer partial views to the reservoir. The campground is shaded by a thick forest of tall ponderosa pine, sugar pine, and white fir, with little understory vegetation. To compensate for the lack of screening, most of the sites are very well spaced.

Lots of pine needles form soft pads for tent pitches, but when walking barefoot, watch out for the small sharp-tipped ponderosa pine cones strewn on the ground, and when setting up your tent or comfy chair, beware of the sugarpine cones falling from above—these cones range from 10 to 24 inches in length, and when one falls nearby you'll sit up and take notice. (If one falls on your tent while you're napping and . . . well, it's better not to ponder this—be proactive.) Some of the sites facing the reservoir are a bit sloped, but each seem to have enough level ground for at least one tent.

RATINGS

Beauty: ✿ ✿ ✿ ✿
Privacy: ✿ ✿ ✿ ✿ ✿
Spaciousness: ✿ ✿ ✿ ✿ ✿
Quiet: ✿ ✿ ✿ ✿
Security: ✿ ✿ ✿ ✿ ✿
Cleanliness: ✿ ✿ ✿ ✿ ✿

The camp hosts set a friendly example by placing a little book-swap station in front of their trailer. With flush toilets and water, Wyandotte is especially welcoming to families, and there are two double family sites with plenty of room for everyone.

Wyandotte opens around Memorial Day, preceding the other larger campgrounds around the lake, and when we camped here in early June, there were still some patches of snow off the sides of Little Grass Valley Road, although the day and night temperatures were wonderfully mild. From the rocky shoreline we plunged into the water, which was cold but warm enough for a short swim—so early in the season, the air was barely hot enough to encourage a longer dip. When we saw boats floating placidly along the lake, we wished for a canoe. Fishing is popular, with the reservoir supporting rainbow trout, German brown, and kokanee salmon. The roar of power boats is occasionally audible from the campground but competes well with the sound of the wind through the trees.

You can hike on a path around the reservoir (it's 13.5 miles all the way around), but for a more scenic hike, you can drive to two nearby trailheads: trek part of the Pacific Crest Trail from the Fowler's Peak trailhead, or hike the Hartman Bar Trail to the Middle Fork of the Feather River. Pick up the Plumas National Forest map from an outdoor retailer to find your way there.

We enjoyed excellent bird-watching right in our campground, observing western tanagers (males are particularly conspicuous yellow-breasted, red-headed birds) in the surrounding trees, and a trio of ospreys (fish hawks) soaring and calling overhead all day long. At night, owls hooted back and forth, and in the morning we rose to coyote howls in the distance.

Once you leave Oroville, the trip to Little Grass Valley Reservoir passes through a series of small towns and settlements, with very few services. La Porte is small and offers limited facilities, most notably a restaurant and tiny general store. Your best bet to stock up on supplies is Oroville, where you can gas up and purchase food and firewood. In La Porte there was no wood for sale in the store, but the town hosts a

KEY INFORMATION

ADDRESS: Feather River Ranger District Plumas National Forest 875 Mitchell Ave. Oroville, CA 95965-4699

OPERATED BY: Northwest Park Management

INFORMATION: (530) 534-6500; www.fs.fed.us/r5/plumas or www.ucampwithus.com/Little Grassarea.html

OPEN: Memorial Day–October

SITES: 34 sites for tents or RVs up to 50 feet; 2 double

EACH SITES HAS: Picnic table and fire ring

ASSIGNMENT: First come, first served; reservations available

REGISTRATION: Self-register at information area in middle of campground; reserve by phone at (877) 444-6777, or online at www.recreation.gov

FACILITIES: Flush toilets, drinking water

PARKING: At individual sites

FEE: $20 single, $35 double

ELEVATION: 5,100 feet

RESTRICTIONS: *Pets:* On leash *Fires:* In established pits or rings only *Alcohol:* No restrictions *Vehicles:* 6 people and 2 vehicles per site maximum *Other:* 14-day stay limit

MAP

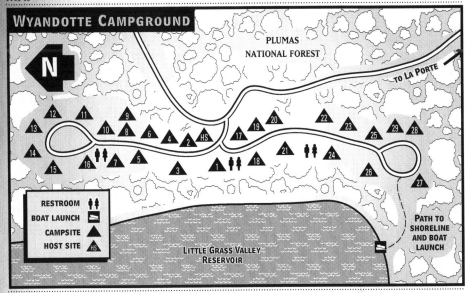

quirky firewood barren of sorts—follow the signs to buy a few armfuls of wood for your campfire.

GETTING THERE

From Oroville on CA 99, take Exit 46, Oroville Dam Road. Drive east 1.7 miles and turn right onto Olive Highway (CA 162). Drive east 6.3 miles and turn right onto Forbestown Road (signed to Forbestown). After 14 miles, continue straight at the Challenge Cut Off, then go 2 miles to a junction with Quincy–La Porte Road. Turn left, toward La Porte. Drive east on Quincy–La Porte Road (FS 120) 24 miles to La Porte. Continue east 2 miles, into Little Grass Valley Reservoir area, to a junction where Quincy–La Porte Road breaks to the right. Continue straight 1 more mile, now on Little Grass Valley Road, and turn right at the sign marked "Peninsula Recreation Facilities." Proceed 0.5 miles, then bear right past the Peninsula Tent Campground, following the small sign to Wyandotte. Continue another 0.3 miles, then turn left into the campground.

GPS COORDINATES

UTM Zone (WGS84) 10S

Easting 0672741

Northing 4399439

Latitude N 39° 43' 38.4634"

Longtitude W 120° 59' 3.7968"

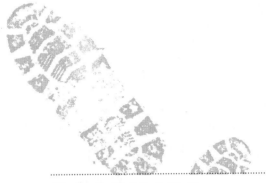

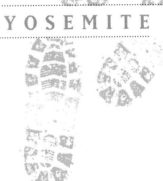

YOSEMITE

ALL ROADS THAT LEAD to Buckeye Campground also pass the Burger Barn in Bridgeport. Anytime is a good time for an everything-on-it burger, wrapped in wax paper, at the outside tables of this ageless monument to roadside dining. Historic Bridgeport's Burger Barn is a famous relic of Americana. One assumes that the lean, tasty burger meat comes from close relatives of the sleek cattle grazing in the knee-deep grass around town. After all, this is cattle country. In Bridgeport, the heart of the Old West steadily beats.

There are four loops to the campground. The first loop you come to on the left, sites 42 through 68, has the campground host (employed by L & L Inc. concessionaires). Bundles of wood are sold at the host station. You continue up the hill for the other three loops. Two have pit toilets, and the other has flush toilets but was closed the last time I was up there.

At 7,000 feet, Buckeye is Big Country camping. The air smells of pine, dust, and cold, rushing water. Buckeye Creek runs right past the campground. The mountain wildflowers grow from the sandy needled floor among the sage. You look up and see the rocky slopes and, farther on, the white of the glaciers on the peaks: it's cowboy country. A horse trail cuts right by the camp. The sites are mostly unoccupied; the pitches are scoured clean by the winter. This is an excellent place to camp.

Fishing is not bad on Buckeye Creek between the two bridges—that's where the fish are stocked. You can hike on over to Twin Lakes and rent a boat. Go for the big brown trout. In 1987 somebody caught the state record holder, a 26.8 pounder, here. However, most of the folks I saw with fish had caught little rainbows. The water-skiing on Upper Twin scares away some of the trout, so the best fishing is on Lower Twin. I talked

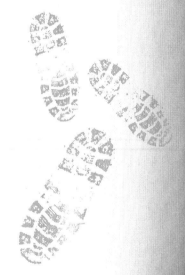

> *Come for fishing, hiking, the magnificent rocky slopes, and far-off glaciers.*

RATINGS

Beauty: ✮ ✮ ✮ ✮ ✮
Privacy: ✮ ✮ ✮ ✮ ✮
Spaciousness: ✮ ✮ ✮ ✮ ✮
Quiet: ✮ ✮ ✮ ✮ ✮
Security: ✮ ✮ ✮ ✮ ✮
Cleanliness: ✮ ✮ ✮ ✮ ✮

ADDRESS: Buckeye
Campground
Humbold–Toiyabe
National Forest
Bridgeport Ranger
Station
HCR 1 Box 1000
Bridgeport, CA
93517

OPERATED BY: U.S. Forest Service

INFORMATION: (775) 331-6444;
www.fs.fed.us/r4/
htnf

OPEN: May–October
(depending on
road and weather
conditions)

SITES: 65 sites

EACH SITE HAS: Picnic table,
fire ring

ASSIGNMENT: First come,
first served; no
reservations

REGISTRATION: At entrance to each
loop

FACILITIES: Flush and vault toilets, drinking water

PARKING: At individual site

FEE: $15

ELEVATION: 7,500 feet

RESTRICTIONS: *Pets:* On leash only
Fires: In fireplace
Alcohol: No
restrictions
Vehicles: RVs up to
30 feet
Other: Don't leave
food out

with one old-timer who said the best time to come for the browns is in May, when it is cold and windy. Troll with rapelas (three- to four-inch minnows), he advised. I threw in some salmon eggs and didn't get a nibble.

Another big draw at Buckeye Campground is the hot springs. They are by the stream down from the campground. It's best to get in your car and drive down the hill. Take your first left and climb a slight hill. There is a slanting parking area immediately on the right. Climb down the steep slope to the hot pools by the river below. This can be fun. Wear shoes with some bite since the footing is slippery. Sometimes the pools are empty, sometimes filled with fun-loving folks. Last time I was there, one pool was occupied by a lone, naked, whalelike chap who looked to me boiled-lobster pink. I chose to wear bathing apparel. I sat first in the hot pool, then sat in Buckeye Creek to cool off.

Good hiking can be had right out of camp. Buck-eye Campground is in a V between the two branches of Buckeye Creek. The two hikes follow the two branches upstream and ultimately swing around and join one another, so you can make up to a 16-mile loop. Bring fishing gear, since there are elusive brown trout and rainbow in the upper reaches; use local worms and try the pools behind beaver dams. The trailhead to the two hikes is up above the campground loops. Just walk up the access road (newly tarred and graveled) and it will dead-end into a horse corral and the trailhead (see the map posted there).

One trail heads west along the right-hand branch of Buckeye Creek. This trail follows an erstwhile wagon road through flowered meadows and pine for-est. The trail up the left-hand branch of Buckeye Creek can be accessed from the campground's left-hand loops (looking west). Just walk to the creek and head up the fisherman's trail. Otherwise, walk from the trail-head a few hundred yards until the trail winds left up a ridge to the stream. The wildflowers in July were all over the place—lupine, shooting star, paintbrush. Watch the campground notice board for ranger wild-flower nature walks—they are fun.

Bring ice—the nearest supplies are at Doc and Al's, or Bridgeport. Think about cooling your beer and

MAP

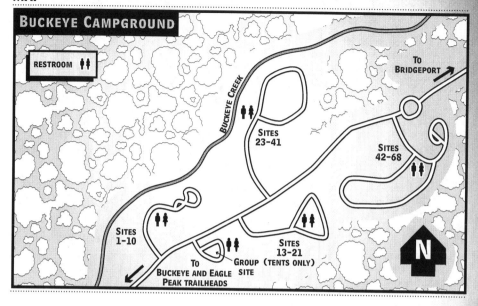

BUCKEYE CAMPGROUND

RESTROOM

BUCKEYE CREEK

TO BRIDGEPORT

SITES 23-41

SITES 42-68

SITES 1-10

SITES 13-21
GROUP (TENTS ONLY)

TO BUCKEYE AND EAGLE PEAK TRAILHEADS SITE

N

sodas in the stream. Or buy a cheap Styrofoam cooler, fill it with ice, duct-tape it shut, and put it in a cool place. Mind the bears. Put all your foodstuff in the car trunk when you go off. Bears are busy tending their cubs and looking for chow during camping season. By fall, bears max out, eating 20,000 calories every day in preparation for hibernation.

Good side trips from Buckeye are to Bodie (bring food and water), Mono Lake, and the Virginia Creek Settlement (once part of Dogtown, a gold-rush mining camp) for a look around and a meal. Go gem-hunting near Bridgeport. Head 3.3 miles north from Bridgeport on CA 182 and turn right on FS 046. Head out exploring but avoid any active mines for quartz crystals, chalcopyrite, and pyrite.

GETTING THERE

From Bridgeport, take the Twin Lakes Road southwest to Buckeye Road on the right by Doc and Al's Resort. Go 4 miles on the dirt road to the campground.

GPS COORDINATES

UTM Zone (WGS84) 11S

Easting 0294497

Northing 4234966

Latitude N 38° 14' 21.2423"

Longtitude W 119° 20' 53.3328"

MINARET FALLS CAMPGROUND

> *The prettiest in a string of beautiful, popular campgrounds on the Upper San Joaquin River.*

MINARET FALLS CAMPGROUND is the prettiest in a string of beautiful, popular campgrounds on the Upper San Joaquin River west of Mammoth Mountain. When you drive down the dirt road into the campground, silvery Minaret Falls leaps out at you. Even in late September, on my last visit, the water cascaded down the mountainside like streams of crystal.

Right away, my wife and I drove into a campsite with a clean and soft tent pitch shrouded by trees. Through the willows we could see the riverbank and the falls.

We drove a few miles up the road to Red's Meadow store and cafe to buy worms and salmon eggs for trout fishing. A little bear was raiding the back room of the store, but the clerk and a tourist scared him away. A dog lunged at the end of his leash, barking at the curious animal as he scurried off. We learned that the original Red was a gold miner who turned to tourism when the Depression and falling gold prices drove him out of business. His pack station at Red's Meadow was one of the first tourist draws in the Mammoth area.

We hiked the 1.25 miles down to Rainbow Falls along with a passel of other folks. We took the rough stairs down to the exquisite falls and stood in the spray. A rainbow arced through the mist.

We hiked back through an area of firs, lodgepoles, and Jeffrey pines, scarred like most of Devil's Postpile National Monument by a 1992 wildfire. Following the fire, rangers walked through the burn to assess the damage, and charred trees crashed down around them. It wasn't safe to walk there for months.

Back at the Minaret Campground we floated salmon eggs and earthworms down the river and caught six trout. My wife wrapped them in aluminum

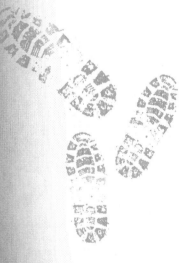

RATINGS

Beauty: ✪ ✪ ✪ ✪ ✪
Privacy: ✪ ✪ ✪
Spaciousness: ✪ ✪ ✪ ✪ ✪
Quiet: ✪ ✪ ✪ ✪ ✪
Security: ✪ ✪ ✪ ✪ ✪
Cleanliness: ✪ ✪ ✪ ✪

foil with herbs and cooked them over the campfire. It was a gorgeous night. The southern Sierras have hundreds of shooting stars.

Sleeping that night in our tent, I heard the rustle of a visitor—a bear. He ran away when I got up. I inspected the damage. My two treasured inflatable Basic Designs sinks, which my wife and I use to wash the dishes, were ruined. The bear had bitten a big hole in each of them. To add insult to injury, he also bit into my plastic collapsible water jug. Were these acts of rancor, or did he think they were full of food?

A neighbor came over. The bear had tried to open the hatch of his Nissan Z; the telltale paw marks gave the intruder away. I told him about my sinks. He recommended wiping sinks, picnic tables, and cooler tops each night with bleach. Bears like soap; bears like everything except bleach. I went back to my sleeping bag and heard the bear slouch through the camp again.

The next morning we walked north along the river and crossed on a log at the end of the campground. There's a short trail to the foot of Minaret Falls. We bushwhacked up to the top of the falls and dipped in some nice pools.

Later, we hiked up to Shadow Lake. It's no easy climb (round-trip is about 7 miles), but you'll agree it's worth it when you see beautiful blue Shadow Lake against huge, craggy Mount Ritter. To find the trailhead, drive back toward Mammoth from the Minaret Falls Campground. Take the road to Agnew Meadows Campground. About 0.3 miles in, you'll find trailhead parking with toilets and drinking water. Follow the signs to Shadow Lake, through another parking lot and across a creek to another trail junction at about 1 mile. To the left is Red's Meadow. To the right is Shadow Lake. With Mammoth Mountain at your back, climb up past Olaine Lake, cross the San Joaquin River on a wooden bridge, and hump it up the canyon wall to Shadow Lake. You'll find good fishing, so bring your fishing gear and bait.

Minaret Falls Campground is popular. Be sure to phone rangers ahead of time to make sure it's open and see how crowded it will be. Try to plan a trip before or after the prime summertime season and arrive on

KEY INFORMATION

ADDRESS:	Minaret Falls Campground Inyo National Forest 351 Pacu Lane Suite 200 Bishop, CA 93514
OPERATED BY:	U.S. Forest Service
INFORMATION:	(760) 873-2400; www .fs.fed.us/r5/inyo
OPEN:	June 15– September 19
SITES:	27
EACH SITE HAS:	Picnic table, fireplace
ASSIGNMENT:	First come, first served; no reservations
REGISTRATION:	At entrance
FACILITIES:	Water, chemical toilets
PARKING:	At site
FEE:	$16
ELEVATION:	7,600 feet
RESTRICTIONS:	*Pets:* On leash only *Fires:* In fireplace *Alcohol:* No restrictions *Vehicles:* RVs up to 22 feet *Other:* No dispersed camping in this area; 14-day stay limit *Note:* To reduce vehicle traffic into the Devil's Postpile area, a shuttle bus system has been implemented. Campers pay a one-time (for duration of stay) fee exemption. Stop at the Mammoth Lakes visitor center (on the right side of CA 203 on the way into Mammoth Lakes) or the Adventure Center (at the ski area) for more information.

MAP

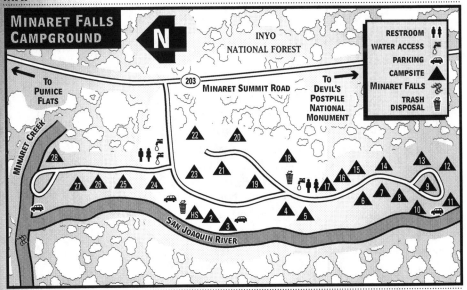

GETTING THERE

Take US 395 to Mammoth Lakes. From Mammoth Lakes, drive 16 miles west on CA 203 (Minaret Summit Road) to the campground.

Thursday if you want to spend the weekend. The area is so popular that during the summer, hikers (not campers) are required to park their cars at the Mammoth Ski Resort and take an intravalley shuttle down.

You have 30 minutes from the time you occupy a campsite to pay. Park your car at the first empty campsite you find, and use that 30 minutes to walk around and see if you like another site better. If you find one, leave something on the picnic table and go move your car.

GPS COORDINATES

UTM Zone (WGS84) 11S
Easting 0316055
Northing 4168050
Latitude N 37° 38' 28.2769"
Longtitude W 119° 5' 5.5465"

48
SADDLEBAG
LAKE CAMPGROUND

Inyo National Forest, east of Yosemite National Park

T**HE SIERRA NEVADA LANDSCAPE** is a pristine and dramatic mix of glacier-carved granite, snow-fed streams and lakes, wildflower-dotted meadows, and ancient forests; this is one of the most beautiful places in the world. At a high alpine elevation, the campground season is short, just a five-month stretch from June (sometimes later) to mid-October. Camping here is like eating the first local strawberries of spring after a winter of tasteless hothouse fruit: intense, sweet, and fleeting. It may spoil you for anyplace else.

Saddlebag Lake is one of five intimate, nonreservable Inyo National Forest campgrounds a mere 2 miles east of the Yosemite National Park entrance station at Tioga Pass. At Tioga Lake, a cluster of open sites sprawl on the lake (but also right off CA 120). Junction Campground, at the intersection of Saddlebag Lake Road and CA 120, is a short distance off both roads but has more trees to provide privacy. Less than a mile east of Saddlebag Lake Road sits Ellery Lake, slightly downhill from CA 120. This campground has some sites well screened by shrubby willows, directly on Lee Vining Creek. Proceeding 1.6 miles up Saddlebag Lake Road, you'll find the easy-to-miss Sawmill Walk-in Campground, on the left. It's a short, level walk to a gorgeous 12-spot campground with well-spaced sites sprinkled across a rocky alpine meadow dotted with pine. At the end of Saddlebag Lake Road sits the crown jewel of the area, Saddlebag Lake, its namesake campground, and trailheads for the 20-lakes basin.

Saddlebag Lake Campground, on a hill above the lake, is reached via a steep gravel road. Although there is plenty of daytime activity down by the lake, the campground is exceptionally quiet. Sites radiate off a single loop, and the ground is somewhat sloped, but gravel tent pads provide level pitches. The premier sites are 16, 18, and 19, which overlook the lake, but

> *Perched on a knoll overlooking one of a series of jewel-like alpine lakes.*

GPS COORDINATES

UTM Zone (WGS84) 11S

Easting 0300323

Northing 4204439

Latitude N 37° 57' 56.2682"

Longtitude W 119° 16' 23.1240"

RATINGS

Beauty: ✩ ✩ ✩ ✩
Privacy: ✩ ✩ ✩
Spaciousness: ✩ ✩ ✩ ✩
Quiet: ✩ ✩ ✩ ✩ ✩
Security: ✩ ✩ ✩ ✩ ✩
Cleanliness: ✩ ✩ ✩ ✩ ✩

ADDRESS: Lee Vining Ranger
Station
Inyo National Forest
P.O. Box 429
Lee Vining, CA 93541

OPERATED BY: Sierra Recreation

INFORMATION: Mono Basin Scenic
Area Visitor Center,
(760) 647-3044

OPEN: June 1–October 15
(weather
permitting); if
planning early- or
late-season camping,
call to be sure the
campground is open

SITES: 20 sites for tents or
RVs (no designated
RV spots, hookups,
or dump station)

EACH SITE HAS: Picnic table, fire
ring, food-storage
locker

ASSIGNMENT: First come, first
served; no
reservations

REGISTRATION: Self-register at
information station

FACILITIES: Drinking water,
vault toilets

PARKING: At individual sites

FEE: $15; if arriving from
the west, $20
entrance fee for
Yosemite National
Park

ELEVATION: 10,087 feet

RESTRICTIONS: *Pets:* Dogs are permitted, on leash during
the day and in your
tent at night
Fires: In designated
fire rings only
Alcohol: No
restrictions
Other: 14-day
stay limit

most of the other sites offer at least partial views to the water as well as the rugged peaks to the north. Spindly lodgepole pines offer only moderate screening between sites, but heck, everyone's looking at the lake anyway.

The lake is actually a dammed reservoir, the water from which flows into Lee Vining Creek and then down to Lee Vining, where it generates power for Southern California. A small cafe squats above Saddle-bag Lake's shoreline, providing simple meals three times a day, small boat rentals, and a water-taxi service across the lake. From the campground it's a five-minute walk to the lake for daylong fishing and hiking adventures. Rainbow trout are stocked, but the lake also holds brook, brown, and golden trout.

The elevation here is more than 10,000 feet, and until you adjust, hiking can be a lung-busting experi-ence. A trail departs from the day-use parking lot, head-ing around the east side of Saddlebag Lake, a less-than-4-mile, nearly level hike. The east leg starts out above the lake, bisecting a sloping hillside where you might see Indian paintbrush and yellow wallflower blooming in summer. Small waterfalls gush downhill into the lake, where even from the trail we could see fish swimming in the clear, sapphire-blue water. The trail gradually passes through a pocket of pines, then approaches the far end of the lake. Here you can extend the 4-mile experience to an 8-mile hike past a series of spectacular alpine lakes. The trail can be hard to follow near Helen and Shamrock lakes, but there is little elevation change to contend with. Back on the west side of Saddlebag Lake, the trail crosses streams and then slips across a talus slope of rocks shed from the mountain on the right. The journey ends near the dam; continue down-hill across the creek to the road, then walk back to the left and up the campground road (the worst hill of the day). If you are really feeling the elevation or don't care to hike at all, take the water taxi ($9 round-trip) from the boat launch near the cafe. The taxi makes explo-ration of the beautiful lakes basin easy.

The cafe sells firewood but not groceries. If you need ice or other supplies, Lee Vining, 12 miles east along Interstate 395, has a few small stores, restaurants,

MAP

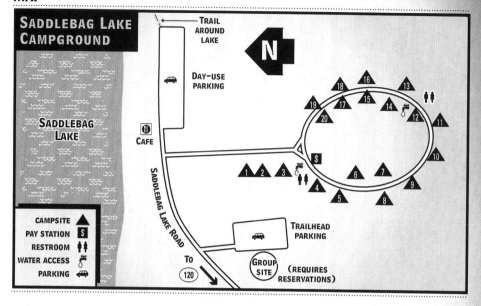

SADDLEBAG LAKE CAMPGROUND

SADDLEBAG LAKE

CAFE

TRAIL AROUND LAKE

N

DAY-USE PARKING

TO 120

SADDLEBAG LAKE ROAD

TRAILHEAD PARKING

GROUP SITE (REQUIRES RESERVATIONS)

CAMPSITE
PAY STATION
RESTROOM
WATER ACCESS
PARKING

and gas. Arriving from the west, the best bet for gas and groceries is the Central Valley town of Oakdale. Once you begin the climb into Yosemite, there are few places to buy food, and gas prices seem to rise with the elevation. Gas is available year-round at Crane Flat and (until early October) at Tuolumne Meadows, but you'll pay a premium. You can also eat in the restaurant at the Tioga Pass Resort (on the north side of CA 120 just west of Saddlebag Lake Road) and buy ice and limited other supplies there.

The campground has food-storage lockers. Use them! At 11:30 p.m. a bear walked past our tent, then overturned a cooler in the adjacent campsite. The bear was run off, but returned at 4 a.m. and ransacked another campsite. We lay in our tent listening to the mayhem. The camp host advises that air horns are particularly effective aids to chase off marauding bears, but the idea of an air horn blast punctuating the quiet of a campground in the middle of the night is less than appealing. For the sake of your fellow campers (and the local bears), keep your food secured in the bear box.

GETTING THERE

From I-5 in San Joaquin County, exit onto CA 120. Drive east on CA 120 through Yosemite National Park ($20 entrance fee). For about 2 miles past the Tioga Pass entrance station, turn left onto Saddlebag Lake Road. Drive north 2 miles on Saddlebag Lake Road (mostly gravel), then turn right at the sign.

From I-395 in Mono County, turn west onto CA 120. Drive west about 11 miles, turn right onto Saddlebag Lake Road. Drive north 2 miles on Saddlebag Lake Road, then turn right into the campground.

> *Don't mind the campground itself. You come for the lakes, the mountains, and the big sky.*

SET DOWN BY THREE TINY jade lakes on the backside of Yosemite, Trumbull Lake Campground is getting popular. It is primitive (no showers), but most of the campsites are reservable. People come back every year. The store in the nearby Virginia Lakes Resort sells beer, ice, and basic supplies. The access road is paved and straight. The fishing is good, the hiking superb. Views of the snowy mountains rising around the three lakes take your breath away. Everybody you meet is complicit, because they are in on the secret that this is the most beautiful spot on earth.

The campground is on a slope above Trumbull Lake. The tiny lake by the Virginia Lakes Resort is over the hill, and the third lake is just a few hundred yards up the gravel road. The campground is like a scruffy dog. You don't like the way it looks, but after a while you learn to love it. The sites are not well engineered. Many are set too close together or too close to the pit toilets—especially the sites down by the lake. You get the feeling the campground evolved haphazardly, but hey, here you are, on the far side of nowhere, pretty close to God.

The drive in is spectacular. Come from Los Angeles and drive up US 395 through the Mojave Desert, the Owens Valley, and up past Mammoth and Mono lakes. This is the most spectacularly diverse terrain in California, with tons of stuff to do on the way. You can also head up from Los Angeles along the west side of the Sierras and come across on CA 120 through Yosemite National Park.

From San Francisco, take CA 108 over the Sonora Pass, where the granite meets the clouds at 9,626 feet. This was the old Sonora and Mono Toll Road, and the men who cut the road had sangfroid. Make sure your flivver is in good shape, and hang on to the steering

RATINGS

Beauty: ☆ ☆ ☆ ☆ ☆
Privacy: ☆ ☆
Spaciousness: ☆ ☆ ☆
Quiet: ☆ ☆ ☆ ☆ ☆
Security: ☆ ☆ ☆ ☆ ☆
Cleanliness: ☆ ☆ ☆ ☆

wheel. It is wild and beautiful—where *For Whom the Bell Tolls* was filmed with Gary Cooper.

I bought salmon eggs and power bait in Lee Vining and caught a decent-sized trout on hooks trimmed off the barb so that I could release (since Tuesday is always spaghetti night). My older sister came along—her first time in the Sierra Nevada for 40 years—and we sat out in the meadow among the lupine and forget-me-nots with a star map and looked up at the sky.

The next day we hiked up to the trailhead by Blue Lake (there's a trail from the campground from site 5 that connects with the trail past the trailhead) and hiked a mile up to Frog Lakes. This is up around 10,000 feet, so expect to suck some air. Take your time and rest often—the older you get, the longer it takes to get acclimated to the rarer air. Then we plugged on to Summit Lake on the Sierra Ridge between Camiaca Peak and Excelsior Mountain to the south. We stopped for sandwiches and soda chilled in the cold lake water, and watched storm clouds close in around Excelsior Mountain (elevation 12,446 feet). We scooted back down to the campground just ahead of a completely unseasonable (early July) thundershower, replete with ear-cracking thunder, hearty gusts of wind, and frightening, white streaks of lightning.

Cringing in our tent under the pines, I regaled my sister with tales of old John Muir, who loved storms and climbed to the top of the highest pine and tied himself in while the elements raged around him, and shouted Walt Whitmanesque exaltations to the primal gods. And John didn't come back to his tent and a towel; he camped in an old overcoat with his sundries in the pockets. He survived one bone-numbing night by crawling into a hot mud spring—alternating cooking one side of himself and freezing the other.

The next morning the sky was as clear blue as the sea, and the chirping sparrows flitted from bush to flower in the meadow. We borrowed an inflatable boat from a camping neighbor and floated around the lake, trailing a little bait and staring up at the mountains above the basin.

I spoke to the campground host (from L & L Inc.), who told me they had plans to make more of the camp-

KEY INFORMATION

ADDRESS:	Trumbull Lake Campground Humboldt–Toiyabe National Forest, Bridgeport Ranger District HCR 1 Box 1000 Bridgeport, CA 93517
OPERATED BY:	U.S. Forest Service
INFORMATION:	(760) 932-7070; www.fs.fed.us/r4/htnf
OPEN:	Mid-June–mid-October (weather permitting)
SITES:	45 sites for tents or RVs
EACH SITE HAS:	Picnic table, fire ring
ASSIGNMENT:	Some sites offer reservations; others are first come, first served
REGISTRATION:	At entrance; reserve by phone, (877) 444-6777, or online, www.reserveusa.com
FACILITIES:	Water, vault toilets
PARKING:	At individual site
FEE:	$11; $9 non-refundable reservation fee; $5 extra vehicle
ELEVATION:	9,500 feet
RESTRICTIONS:	*Pets:* On leash only *Fires:* In fire ring *Alcohol:* No restrictions *Vehicles:* RVs up to 35 feet *Other:* Don't leave food out; no swimming in lake

MAP

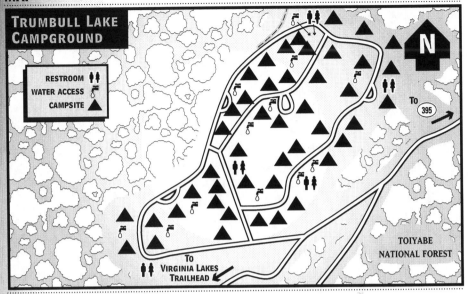

TRUMBULL LAKE CAMPGROUND

RESTROOM
WATER ACCESS
CAMPSITE

N

To
395

TOIYABE
NATIONAL FOREST

To
VIRGINIA LAKES TRAILHEAD

GETTING THERE

From Bridgeport, go about 14 miles south on US 395 to the Conway Summit. Go right (west) on Virginia Lakes Road and drive 6 miles to the campground on the right. From Lee Vining, drive about 12 miles north on US 395 to the Conway Summit and go left (west) on Virginia Lakes Road. Drive 6 miles to the campground on the right.

sites reservable. I checked out all the sites. Sites 10 through 13 are lakeside with a great view but see heavy traffic and are near a pit toilet. I preferred the campsites off the lake, around the fringes of the camp. Site 4 was my favorite. After that came sites 5, 7, 8 (not site 6), and 35 through 37. Still, the campsite itself doesn't really matter. Shortly after arriving at Trumbull Lake Campground, as soon as you take a good look around at the mountains and water, you'll know you're home.

GPS COORDINATES

UTM Zone (WGS84) 11S
Easting 0301816
Northing 4213036
Latitude N 38° 2' 36.1754"
Longtitude W 119° 15' 30.5278"

50
TWIN LAKES CAMPGROUND

THE **TWIN LAKES AROUND THE** Twin Lakes Campground look like blue beans joined at the hip. A little bridge connects the two lakes, and folks in rental rowboats and canoes scoot underneath it. Grandfathers teach their grandchildren how to fish as a waterfall cascades down the cliff above the lakes.

The campground is both accessible and friendly. There are rustic cabins, a lodge, and a store. A few miles away, in the city of Mammoth Lakes, you'll find pizzerias, hardware stores, and a big, wonderful Vons Supermarket on Old Mammoth Road. Twin Lakes Campground is a great place to camp for a week; bring your family for the summer vacation.

The campsites sprawl around the two lakes and uphill across the road. If you find Twin Lakes Campground full, head a few hundred yards up the road to beautiful Coldwater Campground on Coldwater Creek. Or head a mile or so up to Lake Mary Campground and Lake George Campground. All the sites are wonderful but none is reservable. Phone the rangers to check on site availability, and plan your trip so you arrive either in off-season or by Thursday for the weekend.

Head to the top of Coldwater Campground and walk a few hundred yards to the old Mammoth Consolidated Gold Mine on Mineral Hill. Here, you can see some of the old buildings from the mining towns and locations of the many bawdy houses and a saloon named The Temple of Folly (long since destroyed). Walk around the old buildings and rusted machinery and imagine the men who sweated in the summer sun and froze in the winter, obsessed with gold. Climb up to the upper adit in the early morning for a view of Mount Banner and Mount Ritter.

Take the nice little hike to Emerald Lake. It's about a mile up the mountain. The trailhead and parking lot

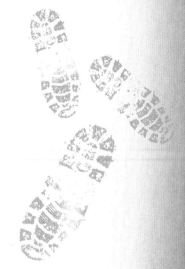

A perfect place to spend summer vacation with the family.

RATINGS

Beauty: ☆ ☆ ☆ ☆ ☆
Privacy: ☆ ☆ ☆ ☆
Spaciousness: ☆ ☆ ☆ ☆ ☆
Quiet: ☆ ☆ ☆
Security: ☆ ☆ ☆ ☆ ☆
Cleanliness: ☆ ☆ ☆ ☆ ☆

ADDRESS: Twin Lakes
Campground
Mammoth Ranger
Station
2500 Main Street
Mammoth Lakes,
CA 93546

OPERATED BY: U.S. Forest Service

INFORMATION: (760) 924-5500; www
.fs.fed.us/r5/inyo

OPEN: May 25–October 31

SITES: 95

EACH SITE HAS: Picnic table,
fireplace

ASSIGNMENT: First come, first
served; no
reservations

REGISTRATION: At entrance

FACILITIES: Water, flush toilets,
boat rental,
wheelchair-
accessible sites

PARKING: At site

FEE: $14

ELEVATION: 8,700 feet

RESTRICTIONS: *Pets:* On leash only
Fires: In fireplaces
Alcohol: No
restrictions
Vehicles: RVs up to
22 feet
Other: To reduce
vehicle traffic into
the Devil's Postpile
area, a shuttle bus
system has been
implemented.
Campers pay a one-
time fee (for duration
of stay) exemption.
Stop at the Mam-
moth Lakes visitor
center (on the right
side of CA 203 on the
way into Mammoth
Lakes) or the Adven-
ture Center (at the
ski area) for more
information.

are next to the parking lot for the mine on Mineral Hill. Walk up by Coldwater Creek where there are lupine, monkey flower, and fireweed. Bring a picnic and climb the rocks around the lake. Bring fishing gear as well. I watched one older woman reel in two decent trout while I ate my sandwich.

If you are ambitious, go around the left side of Emerald Lake. At the signed junction, go right to Gentian Meadow–Sky Meadows. Climb up by the inlet creek and reach tiny Gentian Meadow. Carry on up past a waterfall, and after a while you'll reach Sky Meadows. Look for paintbrush, corn lily, and ele-phant's heads among the grass. It's about 2.5 miles back down the hill.

Or if you are truly ambitious, pick up the trail to Duck Pass (8.2 miles round-trip) back in the parking lot by the trailhead to Emerald Lake. Find the Duck Pass sign and start climbing. When you reach the entry sign for the John Muir Wilderness, bear right. Climb up through lodgepoles, pines, and hemlocks and carry on past the trail to Arrowhead Lake, Skelton Lake, and Barney Lake. Next, you'll see alpine Duck Pass ahead, with all the high-elevation flowers—columbine, gentian, and sorrel. Finally, traverse the pass and you'll see Duck Lake and pretty little Pika Lake on the left.

Back at Twin Lakes Campground, a nice stroll is around the shore to the falls. Access the trail behind campsite 24. You'll see a sign that says "Private Road." Bear left and follow the trail that heads through the trees to the waterfall. Or walk over to Tamarack Lodge. This graceful establishment was built in 1923. The clerk from the grocery store averred that Tama-rack Lodge has the best food in Mammoth Lakes.

However, my wife and I ate chez campsite the last time I was at Twin Lakes. I boiled some quartered pota-toes and set them aside. Then I fried some onions, gar-lic, jalapeño peppers, and strips of chicken breast in the pot. After a bit, I returned the potatoes to the pot and stirred it all about. Very delicious for a one-pot meal!

About 3:15 a.m., I heard a visitor. I jumped out of my sleeping bag and poked my head out of the tent. A three-foot bear was rifling through my cooler of soft drinks. I shouted, and the midget bear looked at me

MAP

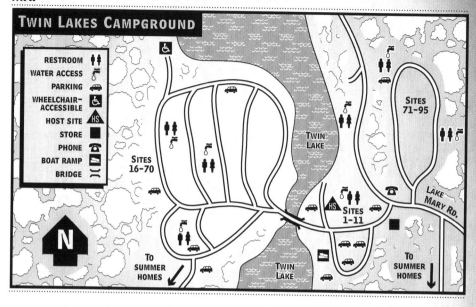

TWIN LAKES CAMPGROUND

RESTROOM	👫
WATER ACCESS	🚰
PARKING	🚗
WHEELCHAIR-ACCESSIBLE	♿
HOST SITE	HS
STORE	■
PHONE	☎
BOAT RAMP	🛶
BRIDGE	)(

SITES 16–70

SITES 71–95

TWIN LAKE

LAKE MARY RD.

SITES 1–11

N

To SUMMER HOMES

TWIN LAKE

To SUMMER HOMES

insolently and pawed on. I threw a pebble, and he ran over to a tree and climbed up a few feet. I retrieved my cooler. He gave me the evil eye and ran into the underbrush. The next morning he was rooting around in the big trash container down by the bridge. He glared at me and sauntered off, combing garbage out of his whiskers.

GETTING THERE

Take US 395 to Mammoth Lakes. From Mammoth Lakes, go west for 3 miles on Lake Mary Road to the campground.

GPS COORDINATES

UTM Zone (WGS84) 11S

Easting 0294069

Northing 4225587

Latitude N 38° 9' 16.8408"

Longtitude W 119° 21' 1.1412"

> *White Wolf Campground is the only campground in Yosemite National Park worth squeezing into.*

YOSEMITE NATIONAL PARK IS HEAVEN on earth. With the Mariposa Battalion, the first English-speaking party to see Yosemite Valley, was Lafayette Bunnell. He wrote: "The grandeur of the scene was softened by the haze that hung over the valley—light as gossamer—and by the clouds which partially dimmed the higher cliffs and mountains. This obscurity of vision merely increased the awe with which I beheld it, and as I looked, a peculiar exalted sensation seemed to fill my whole being, and I found my eyes in tears with emotion."

The Yosemite Native Americans, the original inhabitants, loved the valley too, but the arrival of the forty-niners ended their resiliency. By 1852, Chief Tenaya of the Yosemites, his tribe decimated, was stoned to death by some raiding Mono Native Americans. Soon after, August T. Dowd, a miner hunting in the valley, saw a tree bigger than he'd ever seen before. He told his friends about it, and the tourists began flooding in. Yosemite Valley became a mecca to the world.

Now, four-hour traffic jams in Yosemite Valley are common, and the campgrounds are constantly booked. Avoid Yosemite Valley and explore the rest of the park instead. Come in from the east over the Tioga Pass off US 395 or from the west on CA 120. Shun CA 41, and don't get stuck in the Wawona Tunnel.

However, you should see Tuolumne Meadows and camp in White Wolf Campground. John Muir eloquently described the Tioga Pass area: "From garden to garden, ridge to ridge, I drifted enchanted, now on my knees gazing into the face of a daisy, now climbing again and again among the purple and azure flowers of the hemlocks, now down into the treasuries of the snow, or gazing far over domes and peaks, lakes and woods, and the billowy glaciated fields of the upper Tuolumne. In the midst of such beauty, pierced with its

RATINGS

Beauty: ✩ ✩ ✩ ✩ ✩
Privacy: ✩ ✩ ✩ ✩ ✩
Spaciousness: ✩ ✩ ✩ ✩ ✩
Quiet: ✩ ✩ ✩ ✩ ✩
Security: ✩ ✩ ✩ ✩ ✩
Cleanliness: ✩ ✩ ✩ ✩ ✩

rays, one's body is all one tingling palate. Who wouldn't be a mountaineer! Up here all the world's prizes seem nothing."

White Wolf Campground is full of tiny meadows and stands of lodgepole pine, and the Middle Tuolumne River flows through the campground. The sites are set among the pines and granite boulders. The campground is constructed beautifully; each loop seems miles away from the others. The arrangement of the tables and sites creates a sense of spaciousness. The facilities are clean and well tended. This is slow, elegant camping.

Only the little bear wandering around camp caused a little nervousness. Obviously he was a special bear because he had little colored tags in his ears. Our neighbor shook a towel at the little bear, and he decamped, at least for that day. Of course, we were careful to put away our coolers even if we were only leaving camp for a moment. Bears get a record for raiding campers, and the rangers are forced to take steps. We didn't want that to happen to the little bear with tags in his ears.

We hiked up to Hardin Lake and sat under the pines, reading John Muir. Muir cavorted through these mountains, wearing a great coat and carrying all his gear in his pockets. At night, he lay down in the same massive coat and slept. Those old-timers were real men!

Take John A. "Snowshoe" Thompson, for example. Every winter from 1856 to 1876, Thompson carried the U.S. mail alone across the Sierra. Traveling on skis (called snowshoes in those days), Thompson carried a 100-pound pack and made the 180-mile round-trip in five days. His diet consisted of beef jerky and crackers, and he drank snow. He didn't carry a blanket or wear an overcoat.

At night, Thompson would find a tree stump. After setting fire to the stump, he'd cut some fir boughs for a bed. With his feet to the fire, he'd sleep through the worst blizzards. If he was caught outside camp in a bad blizzard, he just stood on a rock and danced a jig to stay warm.

Today, camping life is a little easier. Still, remember to get supplies in the western flatlands or in Mammoth

KEY INFORMATION

ADDRESS:	Pine Marten Campground Stanislaus National Forest Forest Supervisor 19777 Greenley Road Sonora, CA 95370
OPERATED BY:	U.S. Forest Service
INFORMATION:	(209) 532-3671, (209) 795-1381; www.fs.fed.us/r5/stanislaus
OPEN:	June–October (depending on road and weather conditions); if gate is locked, the grounds are closed; opens after last snow
SITES:	32
EACH SITE HAS:	Picnic table, fireplace, grill
ASSIGNMENT:	First come, first served; no reservations
REGISTRATION:	At entrance
FACILITIES:	Water, flush and vault toilets
PARKING:	At individual site
FEE:	$20
ELEVATION:	7,300 feet
RESTRICTIONS:	*Pets:* On leash only *Fires:* In fireplace *Alcohol:* No restrictions *Vehicles:* RVs up to 22 feet *Other:* Don't leave food out; 14-day stay limit

MAP

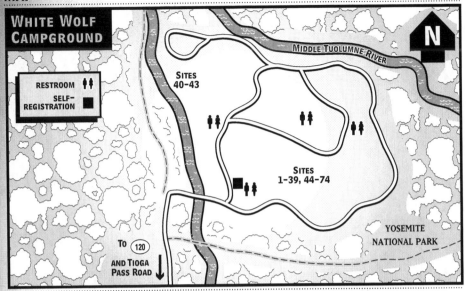

GETTING THERE

Take US 395 to CA 120 (Tioga Pass Road). Go west 43 miles on CA 120 to White Wolf Road on the right. The White Wolf Campground is about a mile down that road.

Lakes on your way in from the east. Only ice, beer, and soda are available in Tuolumne Meadows, Crane Flat, and White Wolf Lodge near White Wolf Campground (in the summer months only).

GPS COORDINATES

UTM Zone (WGS84) 11S

Easting 0267162

Northing 4194776

Latitude N 37° 52' 15"

Longtitude W 119° 38' 50"

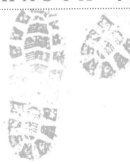

SHASTA-**TRINITY**

52
ANTLERS
CAMGROUND

ANTLERS **C**AMPGROUND **OFFERS ONE** of many opportunities for tent camping around Lake Shasta. It's a favorite of mine for its convenience, great camp host, boat ramp, clean grounds and facilities, and surprising quiet despite being minutes within Interstate 5.

In 1948, Shasta Dam was completed after controversy, a number of deaths, and a delay because of World War II, becoming one of the greatest civil-engineering feats in the world at that time. A curved gravity dam, similiar to the Hoover Dam, it was created as a continuous-pour-concrete project.

When traveling north on I-5, refuel in Redding and stop by the Turtle Bay Exploration Park for further history on the dam and Lake Shasta region. Located beside the internationally acclaimed Sundial Bridge, the park offers information and videos on the dam's construction (among a wide variety of other interesting activities and exhibits for every age).

Shasta Dam changed the entire landscape of Northern California; created hydroelectricity and irrigation for the state; and, let us not forget, formed quite a magnificent lake. The Pit, McCloud, and Sacramento rivers feed Lake Shasta, but only the great Sacramento is released behind the 602-foot-high, 3,469-foot-long concrete wall to flow from Redding through Sacramento and eventually into San Francisco Bay.

I've met a few people who remember the thriving mining towns that were swallowed beneath the lake's depths—517 feet at its deepest—like the town of Kennett, which once had a population of more than 10,000. Lake Shasta also entombed Wintu Indian sacred lands and burial sites, though many of these were moved.

Today, Lake Shasta is a recreation Mecca. There are many exploring options available with 370 miles of

> *The three Shastas—dam, lake, and volcano—are the most dominant forces in this northern country.*

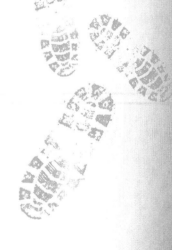

RATINGS

Beauty: ✿ ✿ ✿ ✿
Privacy: ✿ ✿ ✿ ✿
Spaciousness: ✿ ✿ ✿
Quiet: ✿ ✿ ✿ ✿
Security: ✿ ✿ ✿ ✿
Cleanliness: ✿ ✿ ✿ ✿

ADDRESS: USDA Service
Center
Shasta-Trinity
National Forest
3644 Avtech
Parkway
Redding, CA 96002

OPERATED BY: Shasta Recreation
Company and
Forever Resorts

INFORMATION: (530) 275-8113,
www.shastalake
camping.com;
www.fs.fed.us/r5/
shastatrinity

OPEN: Year-round

SITES: 41 sites

EACH SITE HAS: Picnic table,
fireplace, grill,
bear-proof locker

ASSIGNMENT: First come, first
served; reservations
available

REGISTRATION: At entrance;
reservations by
phone, (877) 444-
NRRS, or online,
www.reserveusa.com

FACILITIES: Water, coin-
operated showers,
flush toilets, boat
launch

PARKING: At individual sites

FEE: $18 singles, $30
doubles, $5 extra
vehicle

ELEVATION: 600 feet

RESTRICTIONS: *Pets:* On leash, only
2 pets per campsite
Fires: In fireplace
Alcohol: No
restrictions
Vehicles: RVs to
30 feet
Other: 14-day
stay limit

shoreline. It's the largest man-made reservoir in California and often appears to be several separate lakes when you're cruising up I-5 after finally rising out of the top of the long Sacramento Valley. About 10 miles north of Redding, the highway starts hugging the mountains and then come the sudden glimpses and views of a vast lake.

Antlers Campground is located at the tiny town of Lakehead. Take the Lakehead exit and follow the signs to the east of I-5. Pass the boat-ramp turn-off and then pull into the campground, which is much larger than it first appears. Several loops wind through the tall oaks, firs, and pines.

You won't be lounging on the beach or jumping into the lake from your campsite here. Antlers Campground rests on a cliff above the lake, and depending on water levels, that cliff can be quite significant. There is lake access at the boat ramp and by half-hidden trails, but be careful here. By the way, Lake Shasta doesn't have any beach areas, just plenty of smooth red earth both below and above the surface.

The odd-numbered sites offer the most dramatic views on the lakeside of the campground, but these sites are not for children. The inside sites are perfect for kids, and the pines and tall oaks all around provide beauty and shade from the afternoon heat—this is especially appreciated in July to early September, when the temperatures may reach the triple digits.

The contrast of color on Lake Shasta is striking with vibrant sienna earth and deep-green forests sandwiched between the fluctuating blues of water and sky.

If you'll be boating on the lake or fishing on its edges, you should fill up the gas tank and explore the three river arms that feed Lake Shasta. There's excellent fishing here, with bass tournaments held at various times throughout the year.

The wildlife at Antlers is plentiful—boating friends often tell me they see bears and deer among many other forest critters along the shoreline. We spotted a bald eagle the last time we visited.

Within a 15-minute drive, you can find various other points of interest, including Shasta Caverns; Bridge Bay Marina; and Shasta Dam, which features a

MAP

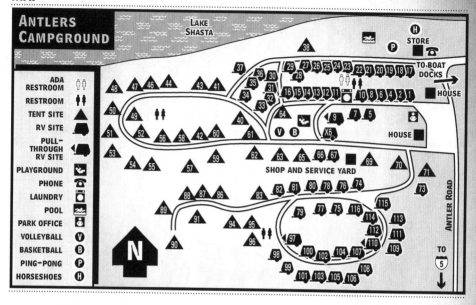

very informative visitor center and the opportunity to walk across the dam.

The three Shastas—dam, lake, and volcano—are the most dominant forces in this northern country, and they will surely satisfy water enthusiasts, mountain lovers, history buffs, or pretty much anyone searching for outdoor excitement.

GETTING THERE

About 10 miles north of Redding on I-5, take Exit 702 to Antlers Road/Lakeshore Drive. Turn right on Antlers Road going north again, and then follow to the campground entrance.

GPS COORDINATES

UTM Zone (WGS84) 10T

Easting 0552347

Northing 4526441

Latitude N 40° 53' 14.5500"

Longtitude W 122° 22' 43.0609"

> *Castle Crags State Park is a paradise for hikers and backpackers.*

JUST **WHEN YOU THINK** the view can't get better going north on 1nterstate 5 from Redding past Lake Shasta, beside the deep gorge of the Upper Sacramento River and toward the mammoth view of 14,000-foot Mount Shasta, around a curve, you catch sight of a remarkable wonder. Out of the forested mountains, you spot a gathering of gray rock spires rising toward the heavens.

This encounter with Castle Crags is most certainly surprising and it warrants further exploration. Luckily for us, a state park here provides abundant opportunities for just that.

Castle Crags State Park is a paradise for hikers, climbers, photographers, and geology lovers. There are 18 miles of trails for backpackers and hikers, with several miles of the Pacific Crest Trail incising the middle. Rock climbers can explore elevations ranging from 2,000 to 6,500 feet; Castle Dome is the most popular rock formation to scale, but only experienced climbers should attempt it. The park also offers excellent camping with all the usual state-park amenities.

But back to the crags. Peering over the ancient trade route called Siskiyou Trail, these granite giants have witnessed some dramatic historical events over the years. One includes the 1855 Battle of Castle Crags, during which poet Joaquin Miller was shot through the cheek with an arrow (he later wrote about the experience in a poem). This battle between Native Americans and gold-rush miners may be the last conflict in the West in which the former relied primarily on bows and arrows. You can guess who won that fight.

Below the crags and hidden within the pines are three loops for camping: Little Loop, Lower Loop, and Upper Loop. Though there are great sites throughout the park, my favorite area is Upper Loop. This section

RATINGS

Beauty: ✿ ✿ ✿ ✿ ✿
Privacy: ✿ ✿ ✿
Spaciousness: ✿ ✿ ✿
Quiet: ✿ ✿ ✿ ✿
Security: ✿ ✿ ✿ ✿ ✿
Cleanliness: ✿ ✿ ✿ ✿

rises up the slope of the mountain, so the walk to the restroom can be a bit of a jaunt in the night, but the sites are level and not too close to one another, the trees are tall, and the peace is palpable. The sites on the outer edge of the loop border the woods, and the western side has a seasonal stream—these are my top picks (within the area includling sites 41 through 64).

Little Loop has only four sites, one of which is reserved for weary hikers coming along the Pacific Crest Trail. This area is also home to the amphitheater where rangers put on demonstrations and movie nights are offered.

Throughout the main campground, the showers are hot and the toilets flush—welcome luxuries after a long day's hike among the crags.

Another option for camping within the park is the Riverside Campground area. If you're traveling north on I-5, turn right after exiting the highway instead of left toward the main entrance of the park. Follow the signs across and parallel to the Upper Sacramento River. Sites 4 through 12 are especially nicely situated along the crystal waters. This river, which becomes the great Sacramento south of Lake Shasta, is a crystal-clear stream running over sand and rounded creek rocks. Take the river trail past the day-use area for great fishing and to find a suspension walking bridge that connects to a trail leading to the main camp-ground (at Lower Loop).

Between the main campground and Riverside Campground are a post office, a gas station where you'll find supplies, and a pay phone. Just several miles north is the historic town of Dunsmuir, which is becoming quite the little artists' community and offers some excellent cuisine—in case you need an evening break from the campfire.

Whether you hike the crags, lounge at your site, or try other outdoor activities in the area, don't miss a short trip up to the vista point. RVs and trailers aren't allowed along the narrow incline, so take the car or use your feet along the trail. And don't forget your camera. From the vista-point parking area, it's a short walk to one of the best views I've encountered—and this is great viewing country. Picnic tables rest at the top of

KEY INFORMATION

ADDRESS: Castle Crags State Park
P.O. Box 80
Castella, CA
96017-0080

OPERATED BY: California State Parks

INFORMATION: (530) 235-2684 or (530)225-2065; www.parks.ca.gov

OPEN: Year-round

SITES: 76 sites, plus 6 environmental sites

EACH SITE HAS: Picnic table, fireplace, bear-proof lockers

ASSIGNMENT: First come, first served; reservations available by phone, (800) 444-7275 or online, www .reserveamerica.com

REGISTRATION: At park entrance

FACILITIES: Water, showers, flush toilets, wheelchair-accessible

PARKING: At individual sites

FEE: $20 ($15 October–May), $7.50 non-refundable cancellation fee

ELEVATION: 2,000 feet

RESTRICTIONS: *Pets:* On leash, not allowed on trails
Fires: In fireplace
Alcohol: No restrictions
Vehicles: 1; RVs allowed; limited space for more vehicles at some sites
Other: Food must be kept in bear-proof storage.

MAP

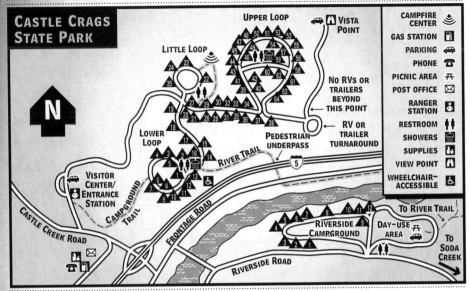

CASTLE CRAGS STATE PARK

UPPER LOOP

LITTLE LOOP

VISTA POINT

LOWER LOOP

PEDESTRIAN UNDERPASS

No RVs OR TRAILERS BEYOND THIS POINT

RV OR TRAILER TURNAROUND

RIVER TRAIL

VISITOR CENTER/ ENTRANCE STATION

CAMPGROUND TRAIL

CASTLE CREEK ROAD

FRONTAGE ROAD

RIVERSIDE CAMPGROUND

DAY-USE AREA

To RIVER TRAIL

To SODA CREEK

RIVERSIDE ROAD

CAMPFIRE CENTER
GAS STATION
PARKING
PHONE
PICNIC AREA
POST OFFICE
RANGER STATION
RESTROOM
SHOWERS
SUPPLIES
VIEW POINT
WHEELCHAIR-ACCESSIBLE

GETTING THERE

Take the Castle Crags exit off Interstate 5, located 6 miles south of Dunsmuir or 50 miles north of Redding.

rise. From three angles, you encounter Mount Shasta, a magnificent direct view of Castle Crags and Castle Dome, and the less beautiful but just as fascinating view of more granite mountains. Bring your lunch or dinner and read about the formation of this region while enjoying a picture-perfect view.

GPS COORDINATES

UTM Zone (WGS84) 10T

Easting 0556806

Northing 4555360

Latitude N 41° 8' 51.2662"

Longtitude W 122° 19' 22.9440"

54
GUMBOOT LAKE AND CASTLE LAKE CAMPGROUND

THE **TOWERING WHITE PEAK** of Mount Shasta stands center stage in far north-central California, gathering attention from every direction and vantage point. And while there are great outdoor opportunities around and on this magnificent sleeping giant, the Shasta-Trinity Forest off its western shoulder holds a treasury of lakes, streams, and glacial formations.

One such treasure is Castle Lake. Famous the world over as UC Davis' Limnological Research Center, it resembles the high alpine lakes of the Swiss and Austrian Alps.

I first visited here as a kid and was awed by this lake unlike any I'd seen before. The water is crystal-clear due to the low levels of plant nutrients in the rocky lake bed. Across the pine-covered shoreline and cut-glass surface rises a mountain of granite, against a clear blue sky. For years, after my first visit, I wondered where that incredible lake resided; happily, I found it again one day while exploring the roads outside Mt. Shasta City. Often a kid's perspective creates disappointment when one revisits an area as an adult, but Castle Lake once again mesmerized me.

Though I've yet to take a kayak onto the 47-acre lake, it's among my top to dos. Seeing rafters and kayakers heading straight out toward the sheer granite face provides a great perspective on just how tall that rock cliff is. The lake is surrounded with fir and pines and offers lakeside trails until smacking into the granite mountain.

Beneath the surface and against the cirque face, the lake drops 110 feet deep, dug out by the formative glaciers of ancient days. At the parking area, the water is less austere at only 10 to 15 feet—you can imagine with such a sharp underwater descent why there's such

> *You've come to one of the most rugged and beautiful areas in California.*

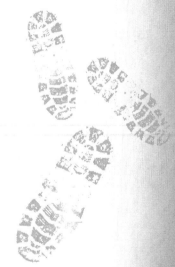

RATINGS

Beauty: ✿ ✿ ✿ ✿ ✿
Privacy: ✿ ✿ ✿ ✿
Spaciousness: ✿ ✿ ✿ ✿
Quiet: ✿ ✿ ✿ ✿ ✿
Security: ✿ ✿ ✿
Cleanliness: ✿ ✿ ✿

KEY INFORMATION

ADDRESS: Shasta-Trinity
National Forest
Mount Shasta Ranger
District
204 West Alma Street
Mount Shasta, CA
96067

OPERATED BY: U.S. Forest Service

INFORMATION: (530) 926 4511;
www.fs.fed.us/r5/
shastatrinity

OPEN: May–October
(weather permitting)

SITES: 6 sites for tents and
RVs (Castle Lake); 8
sites, 4 for tents and
RVs, 4 walk-in across
creek (Gumboot
Lake)

EACH SITE HAS: Picnic table, fire ring

ASSIGNMENT: First come, first
served; no
reservations

REGISTRATION: None

FACILITIES: Vault toilets,
some wheelchair
accessibility

PARKING: At site; parking lot for
walk-in sites

FEE: None

ELEVATION: 5,280 feet Castle
Lake; 6,080 feet
Gumboot Lake

RESTRICTIONS: *Pets:* On leash
Fires: With permit in
fire ring
Alcohol: No
restrictions
Vehicles: RVs up to 16
feet
Other: No motors on
lake; garbage must be
packed out; no drink-
ing water

fascination about exploring the lake within the park's confines.

There's no camping on the lake, but sites are available less than a mile back down the mountain, keeping you close enough for frequent jaunts to the crystal waters, and hiking trails abound throughout the region.

Winter brings visitors to Castle Lake for snowshoe-ing, cross-country skiing, and ice skating, and anglers arrive for some of the best ice fishing around. If you listen carefully, you might catch why a hollow moaning sound led Native Americans to believe that an evil presence inhabited the lake. Today the sound is known to be the ice shifting and the wind roaming the rocky crevasses above the lake.

The Castle Lake area is also known for its vibrant display of red columbine, fawn lily, and Shasta pentste-mon in late spring to early summer. Trails lead into Castle Crags Wilderness Area and on to Castle Crags State Park (see page 177).

Found on the south slope of Mount Eddy, not far along the same ridge of mountains but by way of a longer route by road, is the small but lovely Gumboot Lake. Another alpine treasure, this seven-acre lake offers some wonderful campsites along the water or within view. The area is a haven for nature lovers, with a wide variety of plants, birds, insects, and frogs. Take the informal trail and you might find blue heron near the lake or even bald eagles among the pines and firs.

Fishing is popular here as well. Within my first minutes of arriving at Gumboot, I watched an older couple in a rowboat pulling in a nice trout. Both lakes are stocked, and the fishing can be some of the best around. Rainbow trout, brook trout, and golden shiner are most common. The nearby Gumboot trailhead offers access to the Pacific Crest Trail, and only about 300 feet up a trail is Upper Gumboot Lake.

W. A. Barr Road connects Castle and Gumboot lakes and passes the larger, more developed, and more populated Lake Siskiyou. This is a nice stop for the day if you're in the mood for a refresher on civilization. Motorboats are allowed here ,and boat rentals are

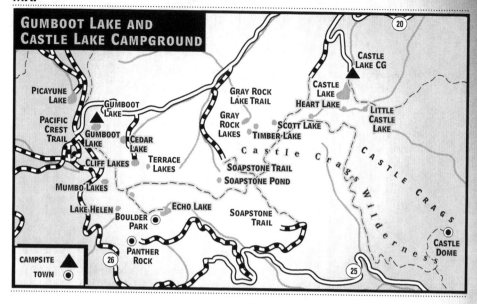

available as well as camping, group sites, fishing, and beaches where you can enjoy the warm afternoons.

Visit Mount Shasta City for shopping, mountain gear, crafts, and art work. The restaurants are diverse, from the Black Bear Diner (offering the best in home-style cooking) to the Billy Goat Tavern (a personal favorite of mine) to a number of ethnic restaurants and natural-food cafes.

However, I highly recommend that you spend the majority of your time as a true explorer of the high country. You've come to one of the most rugged and beautiful areas in California, so explore the roads, trails, and other alpine lakes while staying at or near Gumboot and Castle lakes.

GPS COORDINATES

UTM Zone (WGS84) 10T

Easting 0551955

Northing 4565047

Latitude N 41° 14' 6.5399"

Longtitude W 122° 22' 48.0828"

GETTING THERE

From I-5 in San Joaquin County, exit onto CA 120. Drive east on CA 120 through Yosemite National Park. Take the Central Mount Shasta exit, turn west across the overpass, then south on Old Stage Road, and bear right onto W. A. Barr Road. For Castle Lake, cross Box Canyon Dam, then turn left on Castle Lake Road. Continue on W. A. Barr Road winding around Lake Siskiyou and continuing on FS 26 for 10 miles. Turn left at the fork in the road.

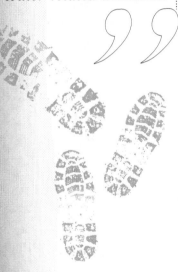

> *With its lovely 36 miles of shoreline and 3,200 acres of surface water, Whiskeytown Lake is a favorite destination for water-related activities.*

NO MATTER HOW MANY TIMES I top the ridge going west on CA 299 from Redding, I'm surprised anew by the serene blue water of Whiskeytown Lake, cupped inside dense pine mountains. It's a sight that makes you want to pause, so pause you should with an immediate left turn at Kennedy Memorial Boulevard and pull into the Whiskeytown visitor center.

President John F. Kennedy made his dedication speech here for the new dam and reservoir in 1963. "I'm proud to be here," JFK said to the attending crowd and the TV viewers who were watching the county's first-ever live television feed. "I congratulate you on what you've done." At the standing box at the far end of the visitor center, you can push a button and hear this speech, which was JFK's last dedication ceremony before his assassination.

Inside the center, you can get current park information, inquire about gold panning and historic mine tours, and view exhibits about the history and development of the Whiskeytown area. Books, maps, and postcards can be purchased in the bookstore.

With its lovely 36 miles of shoreline and 3,200 acres of surface water, Whiskeytown Lake is a favorite destination for water-related activities, and definitely my favorite lake in the area. Even with the massive Lake Shasta a half hour drive to the north, Whiskeytown gathers locals and travelers alike. It has stable water levels, pretty coves, sandy beaches, and convenient marinas.

A lake with above-average clarity (up to 30 feet), Whiskeytown is great for boating, wakeboarding, waterskiing, fishing, kayaking, sailing, and scuba diving. Personal watercraft are no longer allowed, which has curbed the number of accidents and encouraged the popularity of rowing, distance swimming, and

RATINGS

Beauty: ✪ ✪ ✪ ✪ ✪
Privacy: ✪ ✪
Spaciousness: ✪ ✪ ✪
Quiet: ✪ ✪ ✪ ✪ ✪
Security: ✪ ✪ ✪ ✪ ✪
Cleanliness: ✪ ✪ ✪ ✪

kayaking. In the summer, rangers offer guided programs that include free kayak tours.

Reach the best tent camping by continuing on CA 299 west and following the lake to the northwestern end, where you'll find Oak Bottom Marina and Campground. An asphalt section gets dreadfully hot in the summer; not a problem for self-contained RV-ers who are on the lake most of the day, but tent campers should not stay here: temperatures get over 100 degrees in the Redding area during July and August.

Thankfully, some great tent camping is just around the corner, mingled among the pines and close to the cool waters. A wonderful sandy beach area (no lifeguard) offers protected swimming and floating. It's a crescent-shaped cove with beach nearly all the way around. Day-use picnic tables and barbecue grills are available at the back end and opposing peninsula.

On the west side of the beach area is the hilly campground. The best tent sites are lakeside, even with split-level sites dropping down toward the water—there are flat tent and picnic areas at each site. If you've brought or rented a boat (rentals are available at the Oak Bottom Marina), you can tie off just feet from your tent. For plenty of room, choose the upper sites (C-20 through 23, 30, and 33), but my top picks are close to the water for views and refreshing air (A-3, A-7, and the C-section).

Summer is hot here—yes, it's worth saying twice—so spring and autumn are the best seasons for camping on Whiskeytown. The sites at Oak Bottom can get pretty dry from June to September, but with towering pines and crystal waters surrounding, a little dirt won't hurt.

If you do visit during the summer, simply plan your afternoons so that you're out on the lake in a boat or swimming and relaxing at the beach area. After creating some hydroelectricity at the Carr Powerhouse, the Trinity River is the main feed for Whiskeytown Lake. This alpine stream keeps the lake refreshingly cool all summer long unlike some of Northern California's other lakes and rivers.

Trailheads to the region's four waterfalls are within short drives of Oak Bottom Campground. The 220-

KEY INFORMATION

ADDRESS:	14412 Kennedy Memorial Drive Whiskeytown, CA 96095-0188
OPERATED BY:	Forever Resorts, www.whiskeytown marinas.com
INFORMATION:	(530) 359-2269, www.nps.gov
OPEN:	Year-round
SITES:	100 sites
EACH SITE HAS:	Picnic table, fireplace, grill, bear-proof locker
ASSIGNMENT:	First come, first served; reservations by phone (800) 365-CAMP, no reservations for Brandy Creek
REGISTRATION:	At self-registration station, by phone (530) 359-2407
FACILITIES:	Water, coin-operated showers, flush toilets, swim beach, educational programs for kids (Memorial Day–Labor Day)
PARKING:	In parking lot; walk-in to sites (10 feet–500 feet)
FEE:	$18 lakeside, $16 others, $14 RV sites; $13.65 change or cancellation fee; $10 all sites October–May; $5 park fee or $10 for week
ELEVATION:	1,000 feet
RESTRICTIONS:	*Pets:* Not allowed on beach *Fires:* In fireplace *Alcohol:* None allowed in swim-beach area, parking lots, or picnic areas *Vehicles:* Pass required (buy at campground entrance) *Other:* No personal watercraft (such as Jet Skis) on lake

MAP

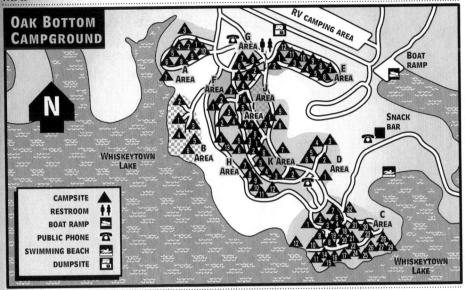

OAK BOTTOM CAMPGROUND

RV CAMPING AREA

BOAT RAMP

SNACK BAR

WHISKEYTOWN LAKE

WHISKEYTOWN LAKE

N

AREA A, B, C, D, E, F, G, H, J, K

CAMPSITE	▲
RESTROOM	👫
BOAT RAMP	
PUBLIC PHONE	☎
SWIMMING BEACH	
DUMPSITE	

GETTING THERE

From Interstate 5, take the CA 44 West exit toward downtown Redding and Eureka. From downtown Redding, follow CA 299 west toward Eureka 12 miles. Turn left at the Oak Bottom Marina and Campground exit.

GPS COORDINATES

UTM Zone (WGS84) 10T

Easting 0462250

Northing 4580747

Latitude N 41° 22' 38.5032"

Longtitude W 123° 27' 5.1985"

foot Whiskeytown Falls has gained international attention being a somewhat new discovery—it was a well-kept secret known only to a few; not even park rangers knew of its presence for more than 40 years. Now with the newly developed Carr Trail, the falls are available for anyone to hike. It's a moderate jaunt, with the trail climbing 700 feet in its 1.5-mile incline.

Brandy Creek Falls and Boulder Creek Falls are other great hiking excursions and are included with Whiskeytown Falls in a stamp card you can get at the visitor center—often some reward is offered for filling all three stamps (such as a poster, or an aquatic-park ticket in Redding). Crystal Falls is also nearby.

If you'll be boating on the lake, take lunch in one of the beautiful coves. My favorite is at the western end at Boulder Creek. It's a perfect spot to swim, relax, and maybe spot deer or bears venturing from the pines to quench their thirst.

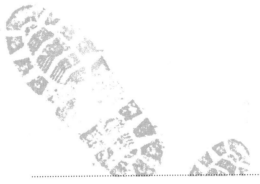

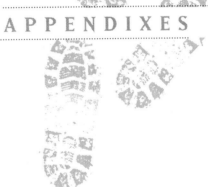

APPENDIXES

APPENDIX A:
CAMPING-EQUIPMENT
CHECKLIST

Except for the large and bulky items on this list, I keep a plastic storage container full of the essentials of car camping so that they're ready to go when I am. I make a last-minute check of the inventory, resupply anything that's low or missing, and away I go!

COOKING UTENSILS
Bottle opener
Bottles of salt, pepper, spices, sugar,
  cooking oil, and maple syrup in water-
  proof, spillproof containers
Can opener
Corkscrew
Cups, plastic or tin
Dish soap (biodegradable),
  sponge, and towel
Flatware
Food of your choice
Frying pan
Fuel for stove
Matches in waterproof container
Plates
Pocketknife
Pot with lid
Spatula
Stove
Tin foil
Wooden spoon

FIRST-AID KIT
Antibiotic cream
Band-Aids®
Diphenhydramine (Benadryl®)
Gauze pads
Ibuprofen or aspirin
Insect repellent
Moleskin®
Snakebite kit
Sunscreen/lip balm
Tape, waterproof adhesive

SLEEPING GEAR
Pillow
Sleeping bag
Sleeping pad, inflatable or insulated
Tent with ground tarp and rainfly

MISCELLANEOUS
Bath soap (biodegradable), washcloth,
  and towel
Camp chair
Candles
Cooler
Deck of cards
Fire starter
Flashlight or headlamp with fresh batteries
Foul-weather clothing (useful year-round in
  higher altitudest)
Paper towels
Plastic zip-top bags
Sunglasses
Toilet paper
Water bottle
Wool blanket

OPTIONAL
Barbecue grill
Binoculars
Field guides on bird, plant, and wildlife
  identification
Fishing rod and tackle
Hatchet
Lantern
Maps (road, topographic, trails, etc.)

APPENDIX B: SUGGESTED READING

Best Short Hikes in California's Northern Sierra. Whitehill, Karen and Terry Whitehill. The Mountaineers, 2003.

California Camping. Stienstra, Tom. Foghorn Press, 2003.

The Complete Poetical Works of Joaquin Miller. Miller, Joaquin. Kessinger Publishing, LLC, 2004.

Easy Camping in Northern California. Stienstra, Tom. Foghorn Press, 1995.

Easy Hiking in Northern California. Brown, Ann Marie. Foghorn Press, 1999.

Gem Trails of Northern California. Mitchell, James R. Gem Guides Book Co., 2003.

Gold! Gold! Petralia, Joseph F. Sierra Outdoor Products Co., 1996.

History of the Sierra Nevada. Farquhar, Francis P. University of California Press, 1965.

Humboldt Redwoods State Park. Rohde, Jerry and Gisela Rohde. Mile & Miles, 1992.

Mendocino Coast. Lorentzen, Bob. Bored Feet Publications, 2003.

Moon Northern California Camping: The Complete Guide to Tent and RV Camping. Stienstra, Tom. Avalon Travel Publishing, 2007.

A Natural History of California. Schoenherr, Allan A. University of California Press, 1995.

Northern California Handbook. Weir, Kim. Moon Publications, Inc., 2000.

Redwood National & State Parks Tales, Trails, & Auto Tours. Rohde, Jerry and Gisela Rohde. Mountain Home Books, 1994.

Roadside Geology of Northern and Central California. Alt, David D. and Donald W. Hyndman. Mountain Press Publishing Co., 2000.

Shasta Lake: Boomtowns and the Building of Shasta Dam (Images of America: California). Rocca, Al. Arcadia Publishing, 2002.

A Treasury of the Sierra Nevada. Reid, Robert Leonard. Wilderness Press, 1983.

Walking California's State Parks. McKinney, John. Olympus Press, 2000.

The World Rushed In. Holliday, J. S. Simon & Schuster, 1981.

APPENDIX C: SOURCES OF INFORMATION

BUREAU OF LAND MANAGEMENT, CALIFORNIA STATE OFFICE
2800 Cottage Way, Suite W1834
Sacramento, CA 95825-1886
(916) 978-4400
www.blm.gov/ca

CALIFORNIA STATE PARKS
P.O. Box 942896
Sacramento, CA 94296
(916) 653-6995
(800) 777-0369
www.parks.ca.gov

ELDORADO NATIONAL FOREST
100 Forni Road
Placerville, CA 95667
(530) 622-5061
www.fs.fed.us/r5/eldorado

HUMBOLDT–TOIYABE NATIONAL FOREST
1200 Franklin Way
Sparks, NV 89431
(775) 331-6444
www.fs.fed.us/r4/htnf

KLAMATH NATIONAL FOREST
1312 Fairlane Road
Yreka, CA 96097-9549
(530) 842-6131
www.fs.fed.us/r5/klamath

LASSEN NATIONAL FOREST
2550 Riverside Drive
Susanville, CA 96130
(530) 257-2151
www.fs.fed.us/r5/lassen

LASSEN VOLCANIC NATIONAL PARK
P.O. Box 100
Mineral, CA 96063
(530) 595-4444
www.nps.gov/lavo

LAVA BEDS NATIONAL MONUMENT
1 Indian Well Headquarters
Tulelake, CA 96134
(530) 667-8100
www.nps.gov/labe

MODOC NATIONAL FOREST
800 West 12th Street
Alturas, CA 96101
(530) 233-5811
www.fs.fed.us/r5/modoc

PACIFIC GAS & ELECTRIC COMPANY
Corporate Real Estate/Recreation
5555 Florin–Perkins Road
Room 100
Sacramento, CA 95826
(916) 386-5164
www.pge.com/about/pge/recreation

APPENDIX C:
SOURCES OF
INFORMATION (continued)

SHASTA-TRINITY NATIONAL FOREST
3644 Avtech Parkway
Redding, CA 96002
(530) 226-2500
www.fs.fed.us/r5/shastatrinity

STANISLAUS NATIONAL FOREST
19777 Greenley Road
Sonora, CA 95370
(209) 532-3671
www.fs.fed.us/r5/stanislaus

TAHOE NATIONAL FOREST
631 Coyote Street
Nevada City, CA 95959
(530) 265-4531
www.fs.fed.us/r5/tahoe

USFS, PACIFIC SOUTHWEST REGION
1323 Club Drive
Vallejo, CA 94592
(707) 562-8737
www.fs.fed.us/r5

INDEX